Veröffentlichungen aus der
Geomedizinischen Forschungsstelle
(Leiter: Professor Dr. Dres. h.c. G. Schettler)
der Heidelberger Akademie der Wissenschaften

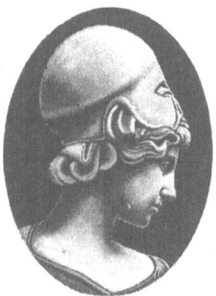

Supplement zu den Sitzungsberichten der
Mathematisch-naturwissenschaftlichen Klasse
Jahrgang 1987

G. Stehle   R. Bernhardt

Coronary Risk Factors in Japan and China

With 23 Figures and 22 Tables

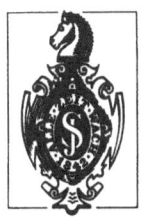

Springer-Verlag
Berlin Heidelberg New York
London Paris Tokyo

Dr. Gerd Stehle
Dr. Ralph Bernhardt

Heidelberger Akademie der Wissenschaften
Geomedizinische Forschungsstelle
Karlstrasse 4, 6900 Heidelberg, FRGermany

ISBN-13:978-3-540-17392-2   e-ISBN-13:978-3-642-82987-1
DOI: 10.1007/978-3-642-82987-1

Typesetting: K+V Fotosatz GmbH, Beerfelden

2125/3140-543210

Contents

List of Contributors

Arab, L., Dr.
Bundesgesundheitsamt Berlin
1000 Berlin, FRGermany

Bernhardt, R., Dr.
Geomedizinische Forschungsstelle der
Heidelberger Akademie der Wissenschaften
Karlstrasse 4, 6900 Heidelberg, FRGermany

Cremer, P., Dr.
Zentrallabor der Universitätsklinik
Robert-Koch-Strasse 40, 3400 Göttingen, FRGermany

Deng, Y., Prof. Dr.
Department of Biochemistry
Tongji University, Medical School
Wuhan, China

Feng, Z., Prof. Dr.
Department of Biochemistry
Tongji University, Medical School
Wuhan, China

Goto, Y., Prof. Dr.
Department of Internal Medicine 1
Tokai University School of Medicine
Bohseidai, Isehara 259-11, Japan

Gross, K., Dipl. Biol.
Geomedizinische Forschungsstelle der
Heidelberger Akademie der Wissenschaften
Karlstrasse 4, 6900 Heidelberg, FRGermany

Cheng, S.
Department of Biochemistry
Tongji University, Medical School
Wuhan, China

Hinohara, S., Dr.
Department of AMHTS
Tokai University School of Medicine
Bohseidai, Isehara 259-11, Japan

Kanemoto, N., Dr.
Department of Internal Medicine 1
Tokai University School of Medicine
Bohseidai, Isehara 259-11, Japan

Schettler, G., Prof. Dr. Dr. h.c. mult.
Geomedizinische Forschungsstelle der
Heidelberger Akademie der Wissenschaften
Karlstrasse 4, 6900 Heidelberg, FRGermany

Seidel, D., Prof. Dr.
Zentrallabor der Universitätsklinik
Robert-Koch-Strasse 40, 3400 Göttingen, FRGermany

Stehle, G., Dr.
Geomedizinische Forschungsstelle der
Heidelberger Akademie der Wissenschaften
Karlstrasse 4, 6900 Heidelberg, FRGermany

Takahashi, T.
Department of AMHTS
Tokai University School of Medicine
Bohseidai, Isehara 259-11, Japan

Tamachi, H., Dr.
Department of Internal Medicine 1
Tokai University School of Medicine
Bohseidai, Isehara 259-11, Japan

Thiery, J., Dr.
Zentrallabor der Universitätsklinik
Robert-Koch-Strasse 40, 3400 Göttingen, FRGermany

Wang, Z.
Department of Biochemistry
Tongji University, Medical School
Wuhan, China

Zeng, J.
Department of Biochemistry
Tongji University, Medical School
Wuhan, China

Blood Lipid Patterns of a Healthy Japanese Population

G. Stehle, S. Hinohara, H. Tamachi, N. Kanemoto, T. Takahashi, K. Gross,
L. Arab, G. Schettler, and Y. Goto

Introduction

Every year coronary heart disease (CHD) claims more than 500000 lives in the
USA alone. In most of the western countries, CHD is after cancer the main cause
of death.

Among the industrialized countries, however, Japan plays a special role. CHD
in Japan is four to ten times less frequent: in 1980, age-standardized mortality
rates of CHD per 100000 persons aged 40–69 were 65 for male and 24 for female
Japanese, versus 398 and 130 in the USA and 630 and 191 in Northern Ireland [1].

Viewed internationally, the prevalence and incidence of CHD are extremely
low in Japan, but viewed nationally, the impression is different, as deaths due to
CHD have increased about fourfold since the 1940s [2].

These epidemiologic constellations provoke interest in the distribution of the
blood lipids in the Japanese population, since high blood lipid concentrations
have been identified as one of a few decisive risk factors intimately associated
with the prevalence and incidence of CHD [3].

Thus, large surveys on lipid concentrations were carried out in Japan in 1960,
1970, and 1980 [4–6]. During these periods, total cholesterol levels increased
gradually but steadily, reflecting the tendency to adopt the western dietary habits
of eating food with a high content of cholesterol and unsaturated fatty acids [2].

To monitor the most recent development in blood lipid levels, we studied the
concentrations of total cholesterol, HDL cholesterol, LDL cholesterol and
triglycerides, as well as body weight, height, and body mass index (BMI) in a free-
living population of 13630 healthy Japanese adults of both sexes.

Material and Methods

In 1984 and 1985, 9479 male and 4151 female healthy Japanese attended the
Automated Multiphasic Health Testing System (AMHTS) of Tokai University
Hospital at Isehara (Kanagawa Prefecture). The city of Isehara (90000 in-
habitants) is located about 50 km southwest of Tokyo and is a typical Japanese

commuter suburb which grew out of a small country town during the postwar period. Health check-ups are recommended for every person 35 years or older in Japan. About 30–40 examinees visit the AMHTS daily. Most of them are sent by their employers as a preventive health care measure [7, 8]. About 75% of the examinees are members of the white collar group and the rest belongs to the blue collar employees.

In the morning, the examinees complete a medical history questionnaire and then given physical and clinical examinations. Physicians instruct the examinees in the afternoon. Blood samples are drawn from the cubital veins into vacuum tubes, with subjects having fasted for at least 12 h before sampling. All blood chemical data are measured immediately afterwards by a SMAC autoanalyzer.

Total cholesterol is determined enzymatically by the Che-Cho-POD (amino-phenazone phenol) method. HDL cholesterol is separated by Mg/dextran sulfate, and triglycerides are analyzed by the Lipase-Gk-PK-LDH method [9].

LDL cholesterol is calculated by the Friedewald formula, excluding persons with triglycerides higher than 400 mg/dl [10]. To adjust for obesity, we used the BMI, which is equivalent to the ratio of the weight in kilograms to the square of the body height in meters. For statistical analysis of the data, we applied the Statistical Analysis System (SAS Institute, Cary, North Carolina, USA).

Results

Total Cholesterol

The serum cholesterol values of all examinees can be described by a curve close to a normal distribution, only slightly skewed to the right.

Mean serum cholesterol concentrations for male Japanese examinees increased with age from 180 mg/dl in the group aged 20–29 to 207 mg/dl in the age group over 70 (Table 1); this is a range of 27 mg/dl, or 15%.

The standard deviations vary from 30 to 37 mg/dl, or from 16% to 18%, from the corresponding mean values not adjusted for age. The lowest cholesterol value measured was 77 mg/dl, the highest 372 mg/dl, these figures encompassing a range of 295 mg/dl.

In female examinees, the mean values for serum cholesterol range from 173 mg/dl to 232 mg/dl, showing a strong age-dependent increase. The lowest and highest mean values are separated by 59 mg/dl, or 34.1%. The standard deviations range from 28 to 43 mg/dl, or from 15% to 18%. Extreme values for the group of female examinees are 95 mg/dl and 437 mg/dl, encompassing a range of 342 mg/dl.

Besides age, sex also plays a major role in the distribution of lipid levels. Young female examinees have somewhat lower levels than their male counterparts. During midlife, women catch up and then overtake men in their cholesterol levels by a considerable 20- to 30-mg/dl margin.

Table 1. Total serum cholesterol levels (mg/dl) of healthy Japanese adults, aged 20–90 Years, by age and sex, sample size, mean, standard deviation, and selected percentiles

MALE EXAMINEES

Age groups	N	Mean	SD	Median	Min	1%	5%	10%	25%	75%	90%	95%	99%	Max
20 – 29	129	180	30	178	95	106	133	144	160	202	216	230	275	277
30 – 34	519	185	34	182	78	120	136	146	163	203	231	246	278	335
35 – 39	1865	193	35	191	96	122	141	151	168	213	238	251	296	338
40 – 44	2680	197	34	194	82	127	145	154	173	218	241	257	289	334
45 – 49	1695	200	35	197	112	129	148	158	176	220	247	263	295	342
50 – 54	1193	200	36	199	77	127	147	156	175	222	247	260	295	372
55 – 59	855	204	37	202	102	126	148	161	178	227	250	266	313	369
60 – 64	295	207	36	204	80	130	152	165	181	231	257	269	292	312
65 – 69	154	204	36	202	103	110	146	161	183	230	248	264	294	298
70 – 90	94	207	35	207	124	129	134	166	180	226	240	259	296	336
20 – 90	9479	197	35	195	77	124	145	154	173	218	243	259	295	372

FEMALES EXAMINEES

Age groups	N	Mean	SD	Median	Min	1%	5%	10%	25%	75%	90%	95%	99%	Max
20 – 29	55	176	28	182	96	98	126	146	161	205	229	242	245	245
30 – 34	203	173	30	170	95	99	128	134	153	193	212	229	257	265
35 – 39	699	185	30	183	107	125	140	147	162	205	225	238	259	297
40 – 44	975	188	30	185	114	129	144	153	166	208	228	240	269	325
45 – 49	775	200	35	197	109	130	147	157	175	220	244	259	299	331
50 – 54	723	217	36	214	123	145	161	172	193	240	266	279	317	361
55 – 59	449	226	38	224	136	149	166	178	201	250	275	290	336	437
60 – 64	185	232	43	235	101	133	165	177	204	253	286	303	354	420
65 – 69	57	231	33	225	147	148	185	191	211	248	273	301	330	330
70 – 90	30	228	31	231	148	150	169	194	217	279	281	299	301	301
20 – 90	4151	201	38	198	95	129	145	155	174	225	250	267	303	437

Table 2. Prevalence (%) of high levels of total cholesterol, HDL cholesterol, LDL cholesterol, triglycerides and high BMI values in male ($n = 9479$) and females examinees[a] ($n = 4151$)

MALE EXAMINEES

Age groups:	N	TOT CHOL (240) %	TOT CHOL (260) %	HDL CHOL (40) %	LDL CHOL (190) %	TRIGLYC (200) %	B M I (26) %
20 – 29	129	3.1	2.3	1.6	1.6	4.7	5.4
30 – 34	519	7.9	2.7	1.5	1.4	15.6	9.1
35 – 39	1865	9.1	3.5	1.3	1.6	16.1	8.0
40 – 44	2680	10.7	4.4	0.9	2.1	17.6	9.1
45 – 49	1695	13.0	5.7	1.1	2.8	21.4	11.3
50 – 54	1193	12.8	5.2	1.2	2.9	20.1	10.6
55 – 59	855	16.1	7.0	1.5	4.3	16.7	10.9
60 – 64	295	16.0	7.8	2.0	4.8	17.3	8.5
65 – 69	154	18.2	6.5	2.0	3.3	7.8	8.4
70 – 90	94	13.3	5.3	2.1	3.2	14.9	7.4
20 – 90	9479	11.6	4.8	1.2	2.5	17.8	9.6

FEMALES EXAMINEES

Age groups:	N	TOT CHOL (240) %	TOT CHOL (260) %	HDL CHOL (40) %	LDL CHOL (190) %	TRIGLYC (200) %	B M I (26) %
20 – 29	55	3.6	0.0	0.0	0.0	1.9	3.8
30 – 34	203	1.5	0.5	0.0	0.0	2.0	4.4
35 – 39	699	4.4	0.9	0.1	0.3	1.2	6.0
40 – 44	975	5.0	1.6	0.0	0.7	1.6	7.5
45 – 49	775	12.6	4.9	0.1	2.3	3.1	10.7
50 – 54	723	25.2	13.4	0.6	6.0	6.4	14.5
55 – 59	449	33.0	16.7	1.3	10.0	8.9	15.6
60 – 64	185	42.2	20.5	2.2	14.1	10.3	11.9
65 – 69	57	38.6	15.8	3.5	7.0	10.5	14.0
70 – 90	30	33.3	26.7	3.3	16.7	16.7	16.7
20 – 90	4151	15.0	6.9	0.5	3.6	4.1	10.1

[a] Included are examinees with total cholesterol levels higher than 240/260 mg/dl, HDL cholesterol less than 40 mg/dl (if total cholesterol higher than 200 mg/dl), LDL cholesterol higher than 190 mg/dl, triglycerides higher than 200 mg/dl, and BMI higher than 26.

Table 3. Correlation coefficients (Spearman) of blood lipids, height, weight, and BMI of healthy Japanese examinees

MALE EXAMINEES

	AGE	TOT CHOL	LDL CHOL[a]	HDL CHOL	TRIGLYC	HEIGHT	WEIGHT	BMI
AGE	--	0.14	0.12	0.02	0.06	-0.29	-0.09	0.08
TOT CHOL	0.14	--	0.89	0.03	0.35	-0.05	0.17	0.22
LDL CHOL	0.12	0.89	--	-0.16	0.18	-0.04	0.16	0.21
HDL CHOL	0.02	0.03	-0.16	--	-0.51	-0.02	-0.28	-0.32
TRIGLYC	0.06	0.35	0.18	-0.51	--	-0.01	0.33	0.39
HEIGHT	-0.29	-0.05	-0.04	-0.02	-0.01	--	0.47	-0.06
WEIGHT	-0.09	0.17	0.16	-0.28	0.33	0.47	--	0.83
BMI	0.08	0.22	0.21	-0.32	0.39	-0.06	0.83	--

[a] $n = 9479$, for LDL cholesterol, $n = 9324$; $r = 0.02$, $p = 0.05$.

FEMALES EXAMINEES

	AGE	TOT CHOL	LDL CHOL[b]	HDL CHOL	TRIGLYC	HEIGHT	WEIGHT	BMI
AGE	--	0.45	0.42	-0.05	0.34	-0.29	0.05	0.23
TOT CHOL	0.45	--	0.92	0.15	0.39	-0.16	0.09	0.20
LDL CHOL	0.42	0.92	--	-0.13	0.35	-0.16	0.14	0.25
HDL CHOL	-0.05	0.15	-0.13	--	-0.40	0.06	-0.23	-0.28
TRIGLYC	0.34	0.39	0.35	-0.40	--	-0.13	0.23	0.32
HEIGHT	-0.29	-0.16	-0.16	0.06	-0.13	--	0.35	-0.17
WEIGHT	0.05	0.09	0.14	-0.23	0.23	0.35	--	0.84
BMI	0.23	0.20	0.25	-0.28	0.32	-0.17	0.84	--

[b] $n = 4151$, for LDL cholesterol, $n = 4140$, all correlations significant with $p = 0.001$.

The prevalence of high cholesterol levels are shown in Table 2. Cholesterol levels of higher than 260 mg/dl can be found in 4.8% of the male examinees (age-dependent range from 2.3% to 7.8%) and in 6.9% of the female examinees (age-dependent range from 0% to 26.7%).

The strong relationship between age and total cholesterol in women is reflected by a correlation coefficient of 0.45, compared with 0.15 in male examinees (Table 3).

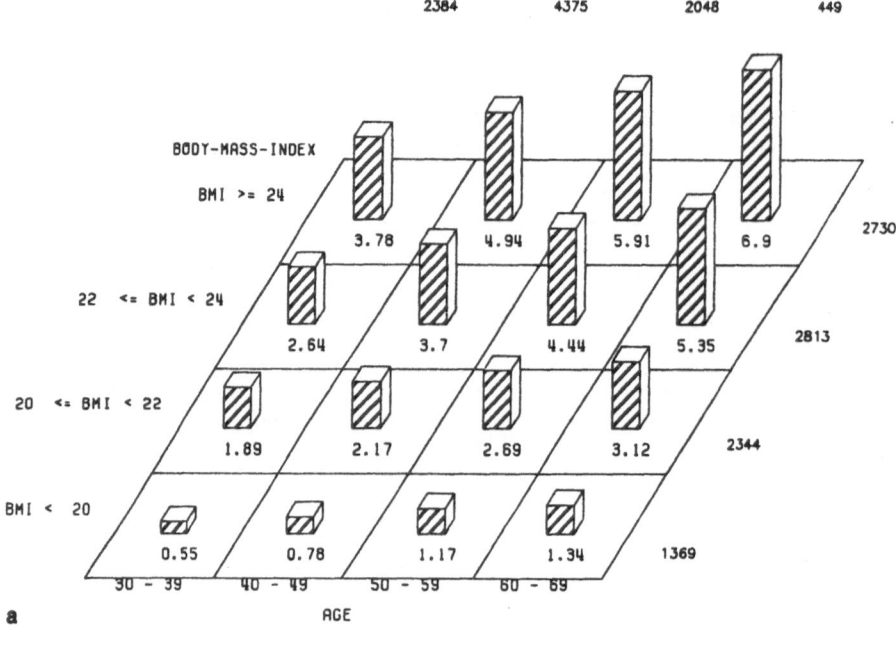

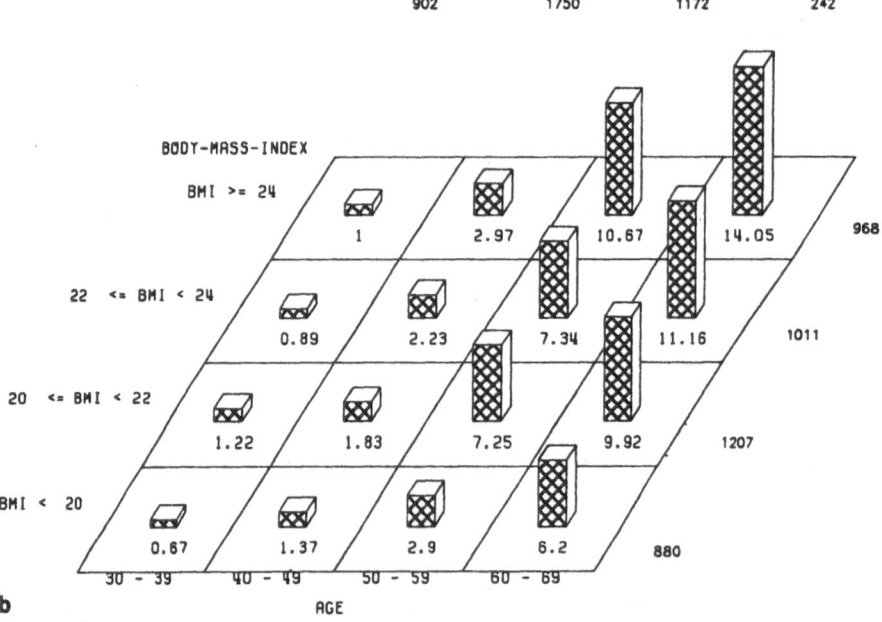

Fig. 1. a Prevalence (%) of hypercholesterolemia (>240 mg/dl) in 9256 healthy Japanese men, adjusted for age and BMI. **b** Prevalence (%) of hypercholesterolemia (>240 mg/dl) in 4066 healthy Japanese women, adjusted for age and BMI

Further positive correlations with total cholesterol concentrations can be found for other lipids, such as for LDL cholesterol (0.89 for male; 0.92 for female) and triglycerides (0.35; 0.39). Both sexes differ considerably for HDL cholesterol, which has correlations of 0.03 for men and 0.15 for women. Body weight and height and BMI also show positive correlations with total cholesterol values (Table 3).

Figure 1 illustrates the influence of age and BMI on cholesterol. In male Japanese, the prevalence of elevated cholesterol concentrations (over 240 mg/dl) shows a five- to sixfold increase, for persons with a high BMI compared with persons with a low BMI.

The effects caused by age are less pronounced: Persons with a high BMI reveal a prevalence of elevated cholesterol concentrations that is two to three times that of persons with a low BMI. For women, a different picture is apparent in Fig. 1 b. The prevalence of elevated cholesterol concentrations is comparatively low in the age groups 30–39 and 40–49 years. For female examinees 50 years or older, a sharp increase (10- to 14-fold) in the prevalence can be observed throughout all BMI classes. In female Japanese, the prevalence of hypercholesterolemia increases by only two- to threefold in persons with a high BMI as compared with persons with a low BMI.

Thus, in Japanese women, age is a more important factor for elevated cholesterol concentrations than BMI, while in male examinees the influence of body weight on total cholesterol prevails over age.

LDL Cholesterol

LDL cholesterol values, as determined by the Friedewald formula, parallel those of total cholesterol, though at levels of about 80 mg/dg less (Table 4).

In male examinees, the lowest mean levels of LDL are 105 mg/dl for the youngest group and rise steadily to 127 mg/dl for the oldest examinees; for the whole group, the mean is 117 mg/dl.

Japanese women show lower concentrations (95 mg/dl) than men for the younger age group, and equal concentrations in the group aged 45–49 (119 mg/dl), which then augment to 145 mg/dl, surpassing levels in men by about 20 mg/dl for comparable age groups.

The prevalence of high LDL cholesterol levels (above 190 mg/dl) show age dependency for both sexes. In male Japanese, the youngest age group shows a prevalence of 1.6%. High LDL cholesterol levels attain a peak of 4.8% for the 60- to 64-year-old examinees, which declines beyond this age to 3.2% (Table 2). In female Japanese below the age of 45 years, elevated LDL cholesterol plays no important role (prevalence 0–0.7%). The turning point comes at the age of 45 years, where the prevalence suddenly increases from 2.3% to 16.7%. Compared with men over 60 years, 3 to 4 times as many women show an elevation of LDL.

The correlations between LDL and other lipid parameters show the same tendency demonstrated above for total cholesterol. There is only one exception:

Table 4. LDL cholesterol levels (mg/dl) of healthy Japanese adults, aged 20–90 years, by age and sex, sample size, mean, standard deviation, and selected percentiles (as calculated by the Friedewald Formula)

MALE EXAMINEES

Age groups	N	Mean	SD	Median	Min	1%	5%	10%	25%	75%	90%	95%	99%	Max
20 – 29	129	105	34	104	42	52	58	67	85	125	143	152	191	211
30 – 34	511	109	29	105	14	52	68	73	89	125	148	169	196	212
35 – 39	1831	113	32	110	19	48	67	76	91	133	154	170	201	268
40 – 44	2638	117	32	115	8	46	69	78	95	136	157	172	199	262
45 – 49	1664	119	32	116	32	52	72	81	97	137	161	178	208	258
50 – 54	1170	118	34	117	15	43	66	77	96	139	160	177	208	333
55 – 59	842	123	35	120	30	54	71	81	98	143	167	187	228	289
60 – 64	291	125	34	123	36	50	74	84	100	147	172	189	212	220
65 – 69	154	125	33	125	47	49	74	81	104	147	170	182	197	201
70 – 90	94	127	37	127	49	55	75	89	94	141	164	177	190	243
20 – 90	9324	117	33	115	8	49	68	78	94	137	159	175	205	333

FEMALES EXAMINEES

Age groups	N	Mean	SD	Median	Min	1%	5%	10%	25%	75%	90%	95%	99%	Max
20 – 29	54	95	25	96	50	58	63	73	87	121	132	155	169	169
30 – 34	202	95	26	93	35	39	57	64	76	112	128	142	164	186
35 – 39	699	107	27	104	39	52	65	74	88	124	139	154	179	270
40 – 44	974	110	27	108	43	56	69	78	91	127	144	158	187	230
45 – 49	774	119	32	117	46	57	73	82	97	138	160	175	218	241
50 – 54	721	133	33	131	55	69	82	92	111	154	178	193	229	269
55 – 59	446	142	36	139	62	67	85	98	119	163	190	203	251	338
60 – 64	184	147	39	145	49	50	86	103	120	168	195	218	265	307
65 – 69	57	144	31	142	68	68	96	111	125	159	179	199	248	248
70 – 90	30	145	44	139	53	60	80	109	127	185	220	221	222	222
20 – 90	4140	120	34	117	35	55	71	80	96	140	165	183	219	338

Table 5. HDL cholesterol levels (mg/dl) of healthy Japanese adults, aged 20–90 years, by age and sex, sample size, mean, standard deviation, and selected percentiles

MALE EXAMINEES

Age groups:	N	Mean	SD	Median	Min	1%	5%	10%	25%	75%	90%	95%	99%	Max
20 – 29	129	54	14	50	30	33	36	39	42	64	76	80	102	102
30 – 34	519	51	12	50	25	30	33	35	42	58	66	72	84	122
35 – 39	1865	52	14	51	14	30	34	37	43	59	70	78	93	129
40 – 44	2680	53	13	51	24	30	34	37	43	60	71	78	90	142
45 – 49	1695	52	14	50	16	29	33	36	42	59	70	77	93	110
50 – 54	1193	53	15	51	17	28	32	36	42	61	74	81	97	115
55 – 59	855	54	16	51	23	28	34	37	43	63	76	85	104	163
60 – 64	295	55	15	53	26	30	34	38	44	63	74	82	105	136
65 – 69	154	55	14	53	23	25	34	37	46	64	75	80	98	99
70 – 90	94	54	16	52	25	27	34	39	44	68	79	84	93	95
20 – 90	9479	53	14	51	14	29	34	37	43	60	71	79	94	163

FEMALES EXAMINEES

Age groups:	N	Mean	SD	Median	Min	1%	5%	10%	25%	75%	90%	95%	99%	Max
20 – 29	55	65	11	66	36	38	45	50	56	74	78	83	85	88
30 – 34	203	63	14	62	26	33	42	48	53	74	82	89	96	105
35 – 39	699	63	14	62	13	36	43	47	54	72	81	87	99	117
40 – 44	975	63	14	62	26	34	42	45	53	72	81	87	101	116
45 – 49	775	63	14	61	26	33	42	46	52	72	82	87	102	115
50 – 54	723	63	16	61	23	32	40	45	52	74	84	92	106	129
55 – 59	449	61	15	58	30	33	39	43	50	70	81	88	103	135
60 – 64	185	61	16	60	32	34	37	40	49	71	83	92	108	124
65 – 69	57	63	15	64	35	37	38	41	52	75	81	89	105	105
70 – 90	30	60	15	65	30	30	34	43	47	72	81	87	88	88
20 – 90	4151	63	15	61	13	34	41	45	52	72	82	88	101	135

LDL and HDL cholesterol display negative correlations for both sexes (-0.16; -0.13)

HDL Cholesterol

Mean HDL cholesterol levels in healthy Japanese men range from 51 to 55 mg/dl (median, 50–53 mg/dl), with a standard deviation of 12–16 mg/dl (Table 5). The extreme values for all men are 14 and 163 mg/dl, the 5%- to 95%-range extends from 34 to 79 mg/dl. HDL levels in the male group remain almost unchanged and independent of age.

In Japanese women as well, no marked variations with increasing age can be described, but it is remarkable that female examinees of all ages have constantly higher HDL levels.

Mean values in women are 60–65 mg/dl (median, 58–65 mg/dl) with a standard deviation of 11–16 mg/dl range, 13–135 mg/dl; 5%–95% interval, 41–88 mg/dl).

The correlation coefficients reveal a minute age effect. However, they show a substantial negative association of HDL cholesterol with triglyceride levels for both male and female examinees (-0.51 and -0.40 respectively), as well as for body weight (-0.28 and -0.23 respectively) and BMI (-0.32 and -0.28 respectively) (Table 3).

Figure 2 demonstrates the prevalence of low HDL concentrations (below 40 mg/dl). The two sexes show different pictures. In male examinees, the prevalence of low HDL concentrations declines slightly with increasing age, whereas this prevalence rises considerably (by eight- to tenfold), the more corpulent men become.

For women, the rates increase significantly only in examinees over 50 years with a high BMI.

If all Japanese with total cholesterol concentrations of below 200 mg/dl are excluded, the prevalence of HDL cholesterol levels below 40 mg/dl drops sharply, ranging in male examinees from 0.9% to 2.1% and in female examinees from 0% to 3.3% (Table 2).

Triglycerides

Triglyceride concentrations are not norm distributed, thus percentiles are to be preferred for description (Table 6).

In young Japanese men, a median of 94 mg/dl for triglycerides has been determined. The median values increase with age, attaining a peak level of 130 mg/dl in the group aged 45–49 and declining subsequently to 107 mg/dl in the oldest examinees (range, 10–969 mg/dl; 5%–95% interval, 51–299 mg/dl).

In women, triglycerides rise with age from 67 mg/dl to 120 mg/dl, exceeding the levels of their male counterparts in the midsixties (range, 10–613 mg/dl; 5%–95% range, 37–190 mg/dl).

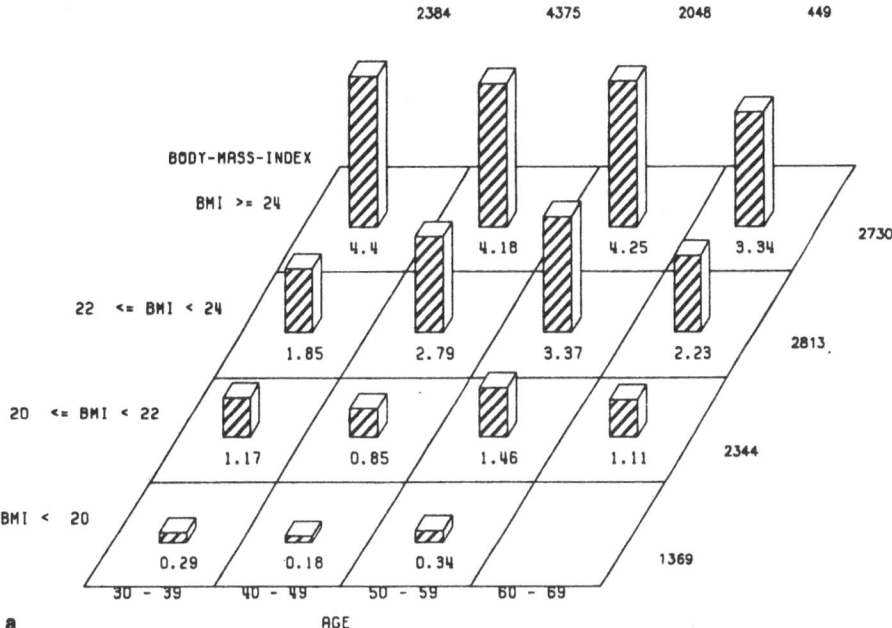

a

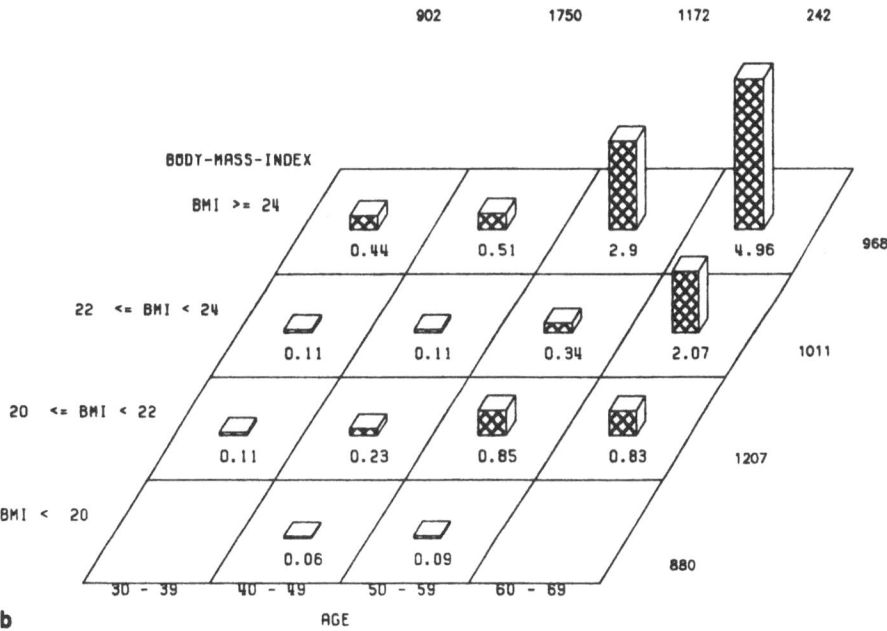

b

Fig. 2. a Prevalence of low HDL cholesterol concentrations (<40 mg/dl) in 9256 healthy Japanese men, if total cholesterol concentrations over 200 mg/dl, age and BMI are considered. **b** Prevalence of low HDL cholesterol concentrations (<40 mg/dl) in 4066 healthy Japanese women, if total cholesterol concentrations over 200 mg/dl, age and BMI are considered

Table 6. Triglyceride concentrations (mg/dl) of healthy Japanese adults, aged 20–90 years, by age and sex, sample size, mean, standard deviation, and selected percentiles

MALE EXAMINEES

Age groups	N	Mean	SD	Median	Min	1%	5%	10%	25%	75%	90%	95%	99%	Max
20 – 29	129	103	46	94	34	36	41	50	74	137	163	194	256	358
30 – 34	519	130	83	102	18	28	43	51	74	160	237	298	454	494
35 – 39	1865	138	89	115	23	34	50	59	81	168	243	301	501	969
40 – 44	2680	140	87	119	17	35	52	61	84	171	241	299	438	922
45 – 49	1695	149	90	130	10	36	54	66	89	186	251	308	487	856
50 – 54	1193	148	89	128	16	40	53	63	89	184	260	309	461	868
55 – 59	855	139	85	121	30	37	51	59	84	168	238	305	424	916
60 – 64	295	137	81	118	35	41	53	62	82	169	241	268	425	694
65 – 69	154	122	54	109	30	33	54	62	82	156	190	227	299	304
70 – 90	94	120	78	112	45	47	55	63	80	183	268	314	321	322
20 – 90	9479	141	87	119	10	36	51	61	84	173	243	299	448	969

FEMALES EXAMINEES

Age groups	N	Mean	SD	Median	Min	1%	5%	10%	25%	75%	90%	95%	99%	Max
20 – 29	55	77	43	67	37	38	39	44	49	91	132	302	551	551
30 – 34	203	72	46	64	20	20	31	35	46	84	119	144	245	467
35 – 39	699	75	41	66	10	24	32	38	50	89	117	142	204	613
40 – 44	975	78	39	69	12	26	35	41	52	93	126	153	222	440
45 – 49	775	89	49	77	14	28	39	45	57	108	147	183	262	522
50 – 54	723	104	59	89	12	31	42	50	65	127	173	218	342	449
55 – 59	449	118	65	103	29	32	45	56	75	144	195	239	351	558
60 – 64	185	121	59	112	31	39	50	60	78	148	203	233	326	431
65 – 69	57	122	66	113	39	39	48	55	79	163	223	286	319	319
70 – 90	30	132	58	120	47	47	50	60	92	177	232	244	247	247
20 – 90	4151	91	53	77	10	27	37	43	56	110	155	190	282	613

Table 7. Body height (cm) of healthy Japanese adults, aged 20–90 years, by age and sex, sample size, mean, standard deviation, and selected percentiles

MALE EXAMINEES

Age groups	N	Mean	SD	Median	Min	1%	5%	10%	25%	75%	90%	95%	99%	Max
20 – 29	129	170	6	170	154	154	160	162	165	174	178	179	183	186
30 – 34	519	169	6	169	150	156	160	162	165	173	176	178	183	187
35 – 39	1865	168	6	168	140	155	159	161	164	172	175	178	182	190
40 – 44	2680	167	6	167	138	153	158	160	163	170	174	176	180	188
45 – 49	1695	166	6	166	149	154	157	159	162	170	173	175	180	184
50 – 54	1193	165	5	165	149	153	156	158	161	168	172	173	177	182
55 – 59	855	164	6	164	144	151	155	157	160	168	171	174	178	183
60 – 64	295	163	6	163	148	149	154	156	159	167	170	173	177	179
65 – 69	154	162	5	162	149	149	154	156	159	166	169	171	174	176
70 – 90	94	161	6	161	143	146	151	154	157	166	169	170	174	174
20 – 90	9479	166	6	166	138	153	157	159	162	170	174	176	180	190

FEMALES EXAMINEES

Age groups	N	Mean	SD	Median	Min	1%	5%	10%	25%	75%	90%	95%	99%	Max
20 – 29	55	158	5	158	143	147	149	151	155	162	164	168	172	172
30 – 34	203	157	5	157	142	142	149	150	153	160	163	164	165	169
35 – 39	699	155	5	156	124	142	147	149	152	159	162	164	167	174
40 – 44	975	155	5	154	137	141	146	148	151	158	161	163	165	177
45 – 49	775	154	5	154	141	144	146	148	151	157	160	162	165	170
50 – 54	723	153	5	153	139	141	144	146	149	156	160	161	164	167
55 – 59	449	152	5	152	136	140	143	145	148	155	158	160	163	164
60 – 64	185	151	5	152	138	140	143	145	148	154	158	160	163	166
65 – 69	57	150	5	151	137	137	140	142	147	154	157	159	162	162
70 – 90	30	150	5	151	136	136	137	143	148	155	156	157	158	158
20 – 90	4151	154	5	154	124	141	145	147	150	157	161	162	165	177

Table 8. Body weight (kg) of healthy Japanese adults, aged 20–90 years, by age and sex, sample size, mean, standard deviation, and selected percentiles

MALE EXAMINEES

Age groups	N	Mean	SD	Median	Min	1%	5%	10%	25%	75%	90%	95%	99%	Max
20 – 29	129	65	10	64	41	47	51	53	57	68	75	80	87	117
30 – 34	519	64	8	63	43	47	51	54	58	69	75	77	88	95
35 – 39	1865	64	8	63	38	46	51	54	58	69	74	79	87	107
40 – 44	2680	63	8	63	34	46	50	53	57	68	73	77	84	92
45 – 49	1695	64	8	63	43	47	51	53	58	69	74	78	84	92
50 – 54	1193	62	8	62	40	45	50	52	57	67	72	75	83	100
55 – 59	855	61	8	61	39	42	49	51	56	66	71	76	82	96
60 – 64	295	60	8	60	41	43	47	49	54	65	71	74	83	88
65 – 69	154	59	8	59	36	38	46	48	54	64	70	73	77	78
70 – 90	94	58	7	58	38	41	43	48	53	63	69	73	76	88
20 – 90	9479	63	8	63	34	45	50	53	57	68	73	77	84	117

FEMALES EXAMINEES

Age groups	N	Mean	SD	Median	Min	1%	5%	10%	25%	75%	90%	95%	99%	Max
20 – 29	55	52	7	51	37	40	41	43	47	56	60	72	73	73
30 – 34	203	51	7	50	39	39	41	43	46	55	59	64	78	84
35 – 39	699	52	7	51	30	37	42	44	48	56	60	64	71	84
40 – 44	975	52	7	52	34	39	42	44	48	56	61	65	72	86
45 – 49	775	53	7	53	38	40	44	46	49	58	62	65	73	86
50 – 54	723	53	7	52	34	38	43	45	49	57	63	66	74	82
55 – 59	449	53	8	52	33	37	41	44	47	58	62	67	73	77
60 – 64	185	52	7	51	36	39	42	43	47	56	60	65	73	82
65 – 69	57	51	8	51	32	32	36	40	45	55	61	67	71	71
70 – 90	30	50	9	50	38	39	39	40	42	55	64	66	74	78
20 – 90	4151	53	7	52	30	38	42	44	48	56	62	65	73	86

The prevalence of hypertriglyceridemia (over 200 mg/dl) shows little influence of age in men (17.8% on an average), but not so in women: their rates increase with age from 1.9% to 16.7%, displaying a correlation of 0.34 (men, 0.06) (Table 3). Another correlation is worthy of mention: HDL cholesterol and triglycerides show factors of −0.51 for men and −0.40 for women.

Body Height, Weight, and BMI

The smallest Japanese man in the group is 138 cm, the tallest, 190 cm. The mean for all men is 166 cm (Table 7).

Mean body height declines by about 1 cm for every 5-year age class, from an initial 170 cm to 161 cm in the examinees aged over 70 years. Women are on an average about 12 cm smaller, beginning with a mean height of 158 cm down to 150 cm.

For men, the mean weight is 62 kg (Table 8). Only three of 9479 Japanese are heavier than 100 kg. For body weight, age dependency can be discerned, with weight decreasing gradually from an average 63 kg in young men to 58 kg in older men.

Female Japanese are about 10 kg lighter than men of the same age, the mean weight being 52 kg (range, 50−53 kg), with no woman heavier than 86 kg. Weight in women is not influenced by age.

Weight and height show a correlation of 0.47 for men and 0.35 for women (Table 3). The BMI shows slightly higher values for men, with 22.6 for men as compared with 21.9 for women (Table 9). While BMI increases with age in women lowest value at 20.2, peak at 22.8, decline to 22.3; correlation, 0.23), the relationship with age in men is less distinct (lowest value at 21.7; peak at 23.0; decline to 22.3; correlation, 0.08).

Discussion

With this primarily descriptive study, we have attempted to give an overview of the actual blood lipid patterns in a Japanese cohort. All 13 630 examinees of both sexes were healthy and free living at the examination date. They took part in the study during a compulsory health check up for employees carried out in 1984 and 1985 at the Automated Multiphasic Health Testing System (AMHTS) of Tokai University Hospital, located in the outskirts of metropolitan Tokyo. The demographic composition of the cohort displays the characteristic profile of suburban Japan: salaried employees, clerks, and other white collar workers accouting for 75% of the examinees; blue collar workers in industry for about 20%; and farmers and fishermen for 5%. For rural Japan, where farmers and fishermen prevail in the population, lower blood lipid levels have been reported before, with serum total cholesterol concentrations that are 10−20 mg/dl lower than those of suburbanites on an average [11, 12].

Table 9. Body mass index (Quetelet Index) of healthy Japanese adults, aged 20−90 years, by age and sex, sample size, mean, standard deviation, and selected percentiles

MALE EXAMINEES

Age groups	N	Mean	SD	Median	Min	1%	5%	10%	25%	75%	90%	95%	99%	Max
20 – 29	129	21.5	2.9	21.6	16.6	16.7	18.2	18.6	19.6	21.7	23.2	25.8	28.3	34.0
30 – 34	519	22.3	2.6	22.1	16.0	17.1	18.5	19.2	20.5	24.0	25.9	27.2	29.2	31.0
35 – 39	1865	22.4	2.6	22.3	15.5	17.1	18.4	19.1	20.7	24.0	25.6	27.0	29.6	34.3
40 – 44	2680	22.6	2.5	22.6	15.8	17.1	18.5	19.3	20.9	24.3	25.9	26.9	28.8	34.2
45 – 49	1695	23.1	2.5	23.0	16.0	17.5	19.0	19.9	21.5	24.7	26.2	27.3	29.5	34.3
50 – 54	1193	22.9	2.6	22.9	16.0	17.1	18.6	19.6	21.2	24.5	26.0	27.0	29.1	33.8
55 – 59	855	22.7	2.7	22.8	15.1	16.5	18.3	19.2	20.9	24.4	26.1	26.9	29.5	34.2
60 – 64	295	22.6	2.6	22.7	16.7	17.0	18.3	19.3	20.6	24.3	25.7	26.9	29.3	32.9
65 – 69	154	22.3	2.7	22.6	15.9	16.0	17.6	18.4	20.5	24.3	25.7	26.8	28.6	28.6
70 – 90	94	22.4	2.6	20.5	16.6	16.7	16.9	18.3	19.1	23.5	29.1	30.3	30.4	30.4
20 – 90	9479	22.7	2.6	22.7	15.1	17.0	18.5	19.4	20.9	24.4	25.9	27.0	29.2	34.3

FEMALES EXAMINEES

Age groups	N	Mean	SD	Median	Min	1%	5%	10%	25%	75%	90%	95%	99%	Max
20 – 29	55	20.3	2.4	20.1	16.0	16.1	16.8	17.1	18.6	22.0	23.2	27.6	28.6	28.6
30 – 34	203	20.7	2.6	20.3	16.1	16.3	17.4	18.0	19.1	21.6	23.6	25.7	30.9	32.5
35 – 39	699	21.5	2.6	21.2	12.2	17.0	18.0	18.7	19.8	22.9	24.8	26.2	29.8	33.1
40 – 44	975	21.9	2.6	21.6	14.2	17.1	18.3	19.0	20.1	23.4	25.2	26.9	29.6	33.6
45 – 49	775	22.5	2.6	22.4	15.9	17.3	18.8	19.4	20.6	24.2	26.2	27.0	30.2	32.3
50 – 54	723	22.8	2.9	22.6	15.3	16.6	18.5	19.3	20.8	24.6	26.8	28.2	31.6	36.2
55 – 59	449	22.9	3.0	22.8	14.6	16.5	18.4	19.3	20.7	24.9	27.0	28.4	30.7	32.3
60 – 64	185	22.7	2.7	22.5	15.5	17.2	18.4	19.0	21.0	24.5	26.2	27.3	29.7	29.8
65 – 69	57	22.5	3.4	22.4	14.2	14.2	15.7	17.5	21.0	25.0	26.4	28.1	31.0	31.0
70 – 90	30	22.4	4.0	22.3	15.7	15.7	16.2	17.7	19.0	24.1	28.0	32.3	34.2	34.2
20 – 90	4151	22.2	2.8	21.9	12.2	16.8	18.2	18.9	20.3	23.8	26.0	27.3	30.3	36.2

In this study, mean values for serum cholesterol were measured, rising age-dependently from 180 to 207 mg/dl in male examinees and from 183 to 235 mg/dl for women. In postmenopausal women, a steep increase of 200–235 mg/dl was observed, such that levels for women surpassed those of men by 30 mg/dl (Table 1).

An age-dependent rise for both men and women, especially those over 50 years, is common for most populations, though at different levels.

LDL cholesterol concentrations paralleled those of total cholesterol, though at a lower level, with an age-dependent rise from 105 to 127 mg/dl in mean values for men and from 95 to 147 mg/dl in women (Table 4).

Sex-dependent differences were obvious for HDL cholesterol concentrations, with women's levels higher by a 10 mg/dl margin (63 mg/dl for women as opposed to 53 mg/dl for men), independently of the age of the examinees (Table 5).

Triglycerides showed sex-specific differences: men had higher levels, with median values starting at 94 mg/dl, attaining a peak of 130 mg/dl at the age of 45–49 years, and then declining to 112 mg/dl.

In young women, triglycerides increase slowly with age. Only for the age groups over 50 years was a steep increase registered, with concentrations ranging from 64 to 77 mg/dl in examinees younger than 50 years and reaching 120 mg/dl in old age. If the correlations between blood lipids, age, and BMI are considered, female Japanese reveal a closer relation of age to total cholesterol, LDL cholesterol, triglycerides, and BMI than male Japanese (Table 3).

HDL cholesterol and triglycerides show a strong inverse relation. The BMI was positively associated in both sexes with serum total cholesterol, LDL cholesterol, and triglycerides, but correlated negatively with HDL cholesterol.

When BMI and age were both taken into account, it was apparent that in men, BMI was the more important factor in relation to the prevalence of high blood lipids than age (Fig. 1–3). However, in women, age was of predominant influence with respect to high blood lipid levels, and only after the age of 50 years did increasing BMI affect lipid concentrations seriously.

Comparisons of these results with those of previous studies carried out in Japan and abroad should be made cautiously because of different analytical and methodological procedures. The racial bias among Japanese and Caucasian Americans has been excluded by the Honolulu Heart Project [13].

Acccordingly, it seems opportune to discuss only the basic tendencies of total cholesterol and HDL cholesterol concentrations in Japan and abroad. About 25 years ago, a large preliminary survey on total cholesterol was carried out, resulting in concentrations ranging from 160 to 190 mg/dl depending on age for both sexes [4]. In the 1970s, studies revealed a gradual and constant upward trend for total cholesterol levels [5,6]. Nowadays, mean values for cholesterol have reached the 200 mg/dl mark in suburban Japanese of either sex. These concentrations are still much lower than those reported for other industrialized countries, where total cholesterol concentrations are 20–40 mg/dl higher [14,15].

Studies of HDL cholesterol levels in health Japanese volunteers, done with the same precipitation technique, measured mean concentrations ranging from 53 to

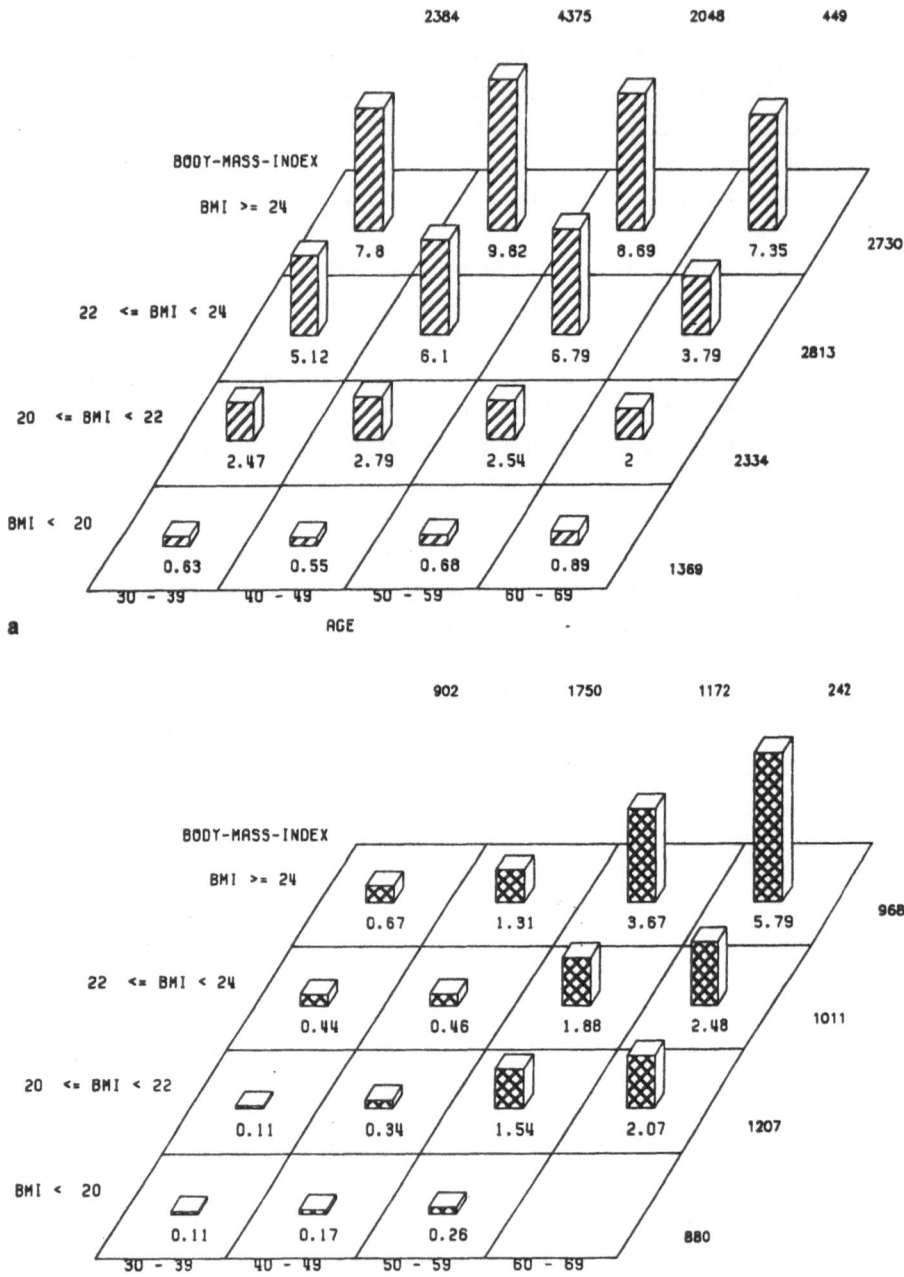

Fig. 3. a Prevalence (%) of hypertriglyceridemia (>200 mg/dl) in 9256 healthy Japanese men, adjusted for age and BMI. **b** Prevalence (%) of hypertriglyceridemia (>200 mg/dl) in 4066 healthy Japanese women, adjusted for age and BMI

Table 10. Comparison of food and energy intake per day
and person in Japan and the USA [20]

products	average food intake in gram	
	(1983)	(1978)
	Japan	U S A
cereals	301	182
rice	202	7
starch/potatoes	92	122
sugar	59	167
vegetables	367	279
fruits	150	206
meat	91	320
eggs	46	45
fish	179	21
dairy products	183	718
fats/oils	41	63
total energy in- intake per day	2 593 KCAL	3 393 KCAL
	10 865 KJ	14 217 KJ

56 mg/dl for men and 61 mg/dl for women [16, 17]. Our results of 53 mg/dl for
men and 63 mg/dl for women confirm these findings, indicating that no decisive
changes in HDL cholesterol levels have taken place during the past decade. HDL
cholesterol concentrations of U.S. Americans and Japanese differ considerably.
For both sexes, HDL concentrations were found to be about 10 mg/dl higher in
Japanese than in Americans [17].

Besides favorable blood lipid concentrations, the Japanese also show a low
prevalence of obesity. For the US population the mean values of the BMI were
calculated to be 25.5 for male and 24.9 for female adults [18].

We calculated indices of 22.7 for male and 21.9 for female Japanese (Table 9).
Thus, major risk factors for CHD, such as blood lipids and adiposity, are less
common in Japan than in the USA.

It is known that these risk factors are dependent on the type of diet consumed
[3]. If the actual nutritional behavior in Japan and the U.S.A. is considered (Table
10), basic differences in diets evolve. Total energy intake for Japanese is 2593 kcal
(10865 KJ) daily, as opposed to 3393 kcal (14217 KJ) for the U.S.A. In addition,
the two nations shows marked distinctions as to dietary composition. Americans

prefer meat, dairy products, and sweets and consume little fish and rice. The average meals of Japanese adults are richer in carbohydrates, especially in rice, vegetables, and high in fish.

However, an alarming change in the Japanese nutritional habits has occurred during the past 25 years. Although the total energy intake has remained stationary at about 2600 kcal (10894 KJ), the intake of animal fat has risen constantly and is now 27 g/day, about three times higher than in 1960 [6]. This development has been parallelled by an increase in serum cholesterol levels [2, 4, 5, 6, 19].

Although conclusions comparing these studies with our results should be drawn cautiously, we feel entitled to state that blood lipid concentrations in the Japanese are still increasing.

A close follow-up of blood lipid levels, especially for young and middle-aged male Japanese, will be necessary in the future. Furthermore, it will be advisable to instruct the populations at risk more effectively on the benefits of adhering to the traditional antiatherosclerotic Japanese diet, instead of adopting a western-style diet associated with a high incidence of CHD.

References

1. Uemura K, Pisa Z (1985) Recent trends in cardiovascular mortality in 27 industrialized countries. World Health Stat Quart 38:142–162
2. Goto Y, Homma Y (1984) Recent trends of coronary heart disease in Japan in relation to dietary alterations. In: Lovenberg W, Yamori Y (eds) Nutritional prevention of cardiovascular disease. Academic, Orlando:73–85
3. Consensus Conference (1985) Lowering blood cholesterol to prevent heart disease. JAMA 253:2080–2086
4. Research Committee on Atherosclerosis in Japan (1965) Total serum cholesterol levels in normal subjects in Japan. Jpn Circ J 29:505–510
5. Research Committee on Hyperlipidemia in Japan (1973) Total serum cholesterol and triglyceride levels in normal subjects in Japan. J Jpn Atheroscler Soc 1:101–113 (in Japanese)
6. Research Committee on Familial Hyperlipidemia in Japan (1983) Changes of serum total cholesterol and triglyceride levels in normal subjects in Japan in the past twenty years. Jpn Circ J 47:1351–1358
7. Hinohara S, Nakadaira S, Takiwaki S, Takahashi T, Suzuki S, Shinozuka T, Hata J, Kawamura N, Noto T, Matsuyama M, Goto Y (1982) Evaluation of usefulness of serial AHMTS. Tokai J Exp Clin Med 7:615–622
8. Hinohara S, Suzuki S, Shinozuka T, Tanabe T, Kanemoto N, Goto Y (1982) Studies on the relationship of cancer detection to check-up intervals. Med Inf 7:179–187
9. Hinohara S, Nakamura T, Takahashi T, Ito K, Shimizu H, Niwa M (1984) Reproducibilities of blood chemical data for AHMTS examinees. Med Inf 9:111–116
10. Friedewald WT, Levy RI, Fredrickson DS (1972) Estimation of the concentration of low-density lipoprotein cholesterol in plasma, without use of the preparative ultracentifuge. Clin Chem 18:499–502

11. Goto Y (1980) Hyperlipidemia and atherosclerosis in Japan. Atherosclerosis 36:341–349
12. Ueshima H, Iida M, Shimamoto M, Konishi M, Tanigaki M, Doi M, Nakanishi N, Takayama Y, Ozawa H, Komachi Y (1982) Dietary intake and serum cholesterol level: their relationship to different lifestyles in several Japanese populations. Circulation 66:519–526
13. Kato H, Tillotson J, Nichman Z, Rhoads GG, Hamilton HB (1973) Epidemiologic studies of coronary heart disease and stroke in Japanese men living in Japan, Hawaii, and California. Am J Epidemiol 97:372–385
14. Abraham S (1978) Total serum cholesterol levels of adults 18–78 years, United States, 1971–1974. Vital and Health Statistics, series 11, no 205. US Department of Health, Education and Welfare, Hyattsville Md
15. Castelli WP, Cooper GR, Doyle JT, Garcia-Palmieri M, Gordon T, Hames C, Hully SB, Kagan A, Kuchmak M, McGee D, Vicic WJ (1977) Distribution of triglyceride and total, LDL, and HDL cholesterol in several populations: a cooperative lipoprotein phenotyping study. J Chron Dis 30:147–169
16. Yano Y, Irie N, Homma Y, Tsushima M, Takeuchi I, Nakaya N, Goto Y (1980) High density lipoprotein cholesterol levels in the Japanese. Atherosclerosis 36:173–181
17. Ueshima H, Iida M, Shimamoto M, Konishi M, Tanigaki M, Nakanishi N, Takayama Y, Ozawa H, Kojima S, Komachi Y (1982) High-density lipoprotein cholesterol levels in Japan. JAMA 247:1985–1987
18. Harlan WR, Hull AL, Schmouder RP, Thompson FE, Larkin FA, Landis RJ (1983) Dietary intake and cardiovascular risk factors. I. Blood pressure correlates: United States, 1971–1974. Vital and Health Statistics, series 11, no 226. US Department of Health, Education and Welfare, Hyattsville Md
19. Ueshima H, Kitada M, Iida M, Tanigaki M, Shimamoto M, Konishi M, Nagano E, Nakanishi N, Takayama Y, Ozawa H, Komachi Y (1982) Serum total cholesterol, triglyceride level, and dietary intake in Japanese students aged 15 years. Am J Epidemiol 116:343–352
20. Japan Institute for Social and Economic Affairs (1985) Japan 1985: an international comparison. Ministry of Agriculture, Forestry, and Fisheries, Tokyo, p. 17

Coronary Risk Factors in China: A Comparative Study of Middle-aged Workers in China and Germany

R. Bernhardt, Z. Feng, Y. Deng, Z. Wang, J. Zeng, S. Cheng, P. Cremer, J. Thiery, D. Seidel, and G. Schettler

Introduction

Cardiovascular diseases are the most common causes of death in both Germany and other Western industrialized nations. They are currently responsible for about 50% of all deaths and therefore contribute more to the death rate than cancer [1]. One-third of all the deaths caused by cardiovascular diseases result from coronary heart disease and resulting heart attacks. Numerous epidemiologic investigations have demonstrated that there are specific risk factors for the development of atherosclerosis. The following list ranks the most potent factors associated with coronary heart disease and heart attacks:

1. Hyper- and dyslipoproteinemias
2. Cigarette smoking
3. High blood pressure
4. Diabetes mellitus
5. Increased uric acid levels
6. Obesity

These factors often occur in combination and thus have a synergistic effect on total risk. In hyper- and dyslipoproteinemias, elevated serum cholesterol levels represent the most important risk factor [2]. Numerous epidemiologic studies, as well as animal and biochemical studies, have revealed that high levels of low-density lipoprotein (LDL) one of the physiologic transport forms of cholesterol, are particularly responsible for the increased occurrence of atherosclerosis. On the other hand, it has been demonstrated that increased high-density lipoprotein (HDL) cholesterol represents a lower risk for cardiovascular diseases [3]. A comparative study on the causes of death in China [4] and Germany [1] revealed that mortality from myocardial infarction and ischemic heart disease is much lower in China than in Germany (Table 1). This finding may be an important contribution toward accounting for the fact that life expectancy in China is nearly as long as in Western countries [5] (Table 2), although the Chinese health care system needs substantial inprovements, especially in rural regions. Severe infectious diseases like hepatitis and tuberculosis play an important role in mortality statistics in China.

Table 1. Causes of death (%) in 1982

	China	FRG [1]
Myocardial infarction and other chemic heart diseases	5.8	18.4
Cerebrovascular diseases	26.8	13.9
Other cardiovascular diseases	11.5	18.0
Cancer	21.4	21.1
Accidents and suicides	14.6	.4
Other diseases	19.9	25.2

Table 2. Average life expectancy of newborn (years)

	Men	Women
China 1978 [5]	69.4	73.2
Country	66.7	69.2
Total	67.0	70.0
FRG 1979 – 1981 [1]	69.9	76.6
USA 1980 [1]	70.0	77.6
Japan 1980 [1]	73.3	78.8

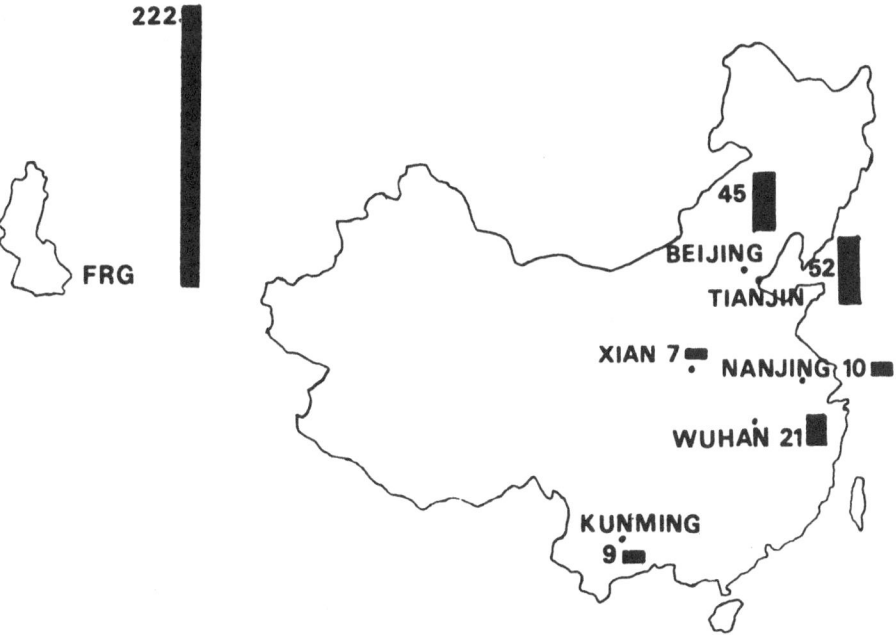

Fig. 1. Mortality due to coronary heart disease in 1977 (1:100000)

Figure 1 shows that in respect to the mortality rate of coronary heart disease, there is a North-South pattern in China similar to that in Europe. However, the higher rate of death in the northern part of China is still lower than that occurring in Germany.

Some Chinese publications [6] suggest that lower serum cholesterol levels are probably the reason for lower rates of heart attacks in the Chinese population. However, the results of those studies cannot be accurately compared with data from Western countries because the groups and methods differ. A recent publication compared serum lipid levels of people in Beijing and Belgium under identical laboratory conditions [7]. The present study, however, represents the first study of the complete cardiovascular risk factor profile in China conducted under investigative methods similar to those used in a German study. Follow-up investigations of both groups 5 years after the initial contact are planned. In these, differences in morbidity and mortality between the two countries and changes in the risk factors due to increasing industrialization in China will need to be taken into account.

Methods

Data

From 12 March 1982 to 6 September 1983, 2146 male laborers and employers were chosen from seven specific factories and examined. The participation rate in the 40- to 60-year-old age range was 76%. The investigation program included a personal and family history, a physical examination including electrocardiogram (ECG), blood pressure measurement, body weight determination, a semiquantitative determination of protein and glucose in urine, and the collection of 10 ml venous blood taken at least 12 h after the last meal. The questionnaire included 53 questions following the form of the 1982 Göttingen Risk, Incidence, and Prevalence Study (GRIPS) [8].

Laboratory Methods

As far as possible, the methods used in the GRIPS were employed. The blood sample was centrifuged 60 min after the blood was withdrawn and analyzed within the next 36 h. A portion of each serum sample was frozen immediately at $-70\,^\circ$C and transported to Germany for determination of the apoproteins. The lipoproteins were stabilized by the addition of saccharose to a final concentration of 20% before the samples were frozen. The determination of cholesterol, triglycerides, uric acid, glucose, creatinine, glutamate pyruvate transaminase (GPT), gamma-glutamyl transpeptidase (gamma-GT), and alkaline phosphatase levels were performed with test materials from Boehringer Mannheim. The cholesterol was measured according to the CHOD-PAP method [10]. The apolipoproteins were determined by kinetic nephelometry [11, 12].

The lipoprotein fractions were measured by quantitative lipoprotein elec-trophoresis, followed by polyanion precipitation densitometry [13]. Additional methods included the measurement of HDL cholesterol in the supernatant after precipitation with phosphotungstate acid (Boehringer Mannheim) [14], as well as with heparin (Merck, Darmstadt) [15]. LDL cholesterol was estimated according to the Friedewald formula [16] and measured separately by a method [19] whereby heparin at pH 5.12 selectively precipitates LDL (Merck, Darmstadt). All photometry measurements were performed on an Eppendorf photometer PCP 6121.

Statistical Analysis

The cumulative frequency distributions of investigative results are graphically presented showing the percentage of subjects greater or equal to a certain value of the parameter. The remaining statistical evaluations were performed using the SAS systems [17].

Nutritional Evaluation

A random sample study consisting of 262 participants was performed using the 24-h recall protocol. In this study, the number of participants for each week day was constant. Available nutritional intake was evaluated from Chinese food com-position tables.

Results

Age distribution (Fig. 2) within the evaluated group of men 40−60 years old shows the predominance of the younger age group, explained by the early retire-ment of many of the older age groups. The German group showed a similar, though less specific age difference distribution. However, the parameters in-vestigated in those studies demonstrate little age dependence (Table 3). Cigarette consumption (Fig. 3) in the male Chinese population was demonstrably higher than in Germany. The Chinese government has only recently begun to educate the public that cigarette smoking is damaging to health and should be reduced. That the proportion of exsmokers in China is lower than in Germany may be at-tributable to this. Lower alcohol consumption (Fig. 4) is reported for more than half of the Chinese male population. Heavy drinkers are relatively seldom; 95% of the Chinese population sample consumed no more than 40 g/day alcohol. The gamma-GT measurements also showed 95% of the sample population to be within the normal range of up to 28 U/ml (Fig. 5). No significant differences be-tween the Chinese and the German group were found with respect to alkaline phosphatase activity (Fig. 6).

A considerable amount of physical activity is common to all Chinese laborers, since they usually travel daily from home to the job by walking or by bicycle.

Fig. 2. Age distribution (years)

	Wuhan	Göttingen
Descriptive statistics		
Mean	46.8	47.7
Median	46	46.8
Standard deviation	5.0	5.3
5.–95. percentile	40–56	40.7–56.8
Minimum-maximum	40–60	40–60
Correlations (Pearson correlation coefficients for $p<0.01$)		
Broca index	pos. (0.11)	
Blood pressure	pos. (0.20)	
Heart rate	n.s.	
Cigarette consumption	neg. (−0.08)	
Alcohol consumption	pos. (0.07)	
Alkaline phosphatase	n.s.	
Gamma-GT	pos. (0.07)	
GPT	n.s.	
Triglycerides	n.s.	
Cholesterol	pos. (0.11)	
HDL cholesterol	pos. (0.07)	
LDL cholesterol	pos. (0.10)	
VLDL cholesterol	n.s.	
Ratio LDL/HDL	n.s.	
Uric acid	pos. (0.07)	
Glucose	pos. (0.09)	

Cumulative frequency distribution

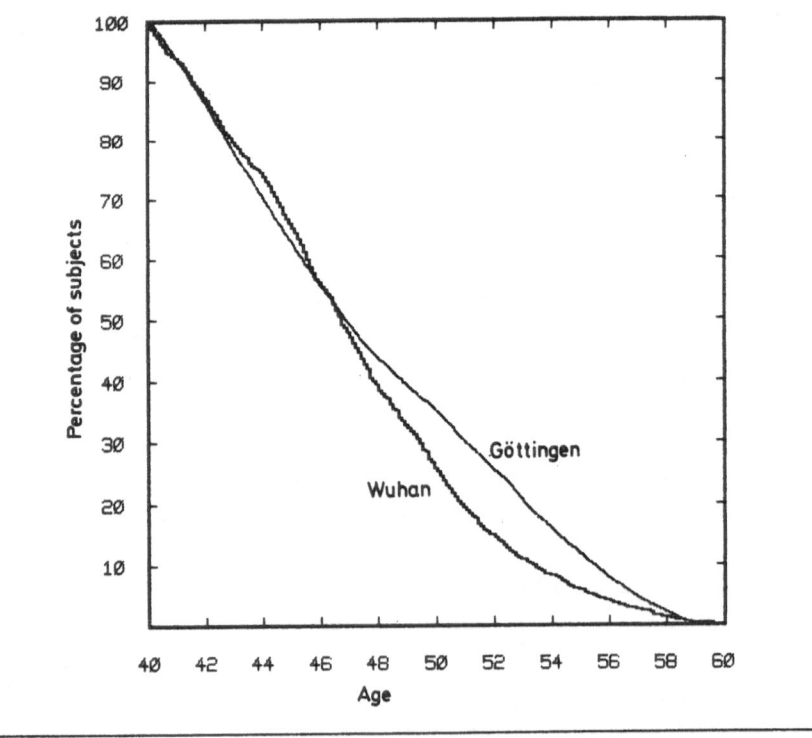

Table 3. Influence of age

	41 – 45 years	46 – 50 years	51 – 55 years	56 – 60 years
(*n*)	572	822	409	121
Broca index (%)	88.2	88.9	90.8	92.6
Blood pressure, systolic (mmHg)	117	120	124	135
Blood pressure, diastolic (mmHg)	76	77	80	84
Triglycerides (mg/dl)	113	117	119	112
Cholesterol (mg/dl)	150	157	157	162
HDL cholesterol (mg/dl)	48.1	50.0	49.6	51.7
LDL cholesterol (mg/dl)	91.0	95.7	96.0	101.0
VLDL cholesterol (mg/dl)	11.1	11.1	11.3	10.0
Uric acid (mg/dl)	4.7	4.7	4.7	4.9
Glucose (mg/dl)	85	87	87	94

Table 4. Case history of earlier or present diseases

	(*n*)	(%)
Diseases of the gastrointestinal tract	356	16.6
Hepatitis	329	15.3
Other liver diseases	36	1.7
Lung tuberculosis	121	5.6
Other lung diseases	139	6.5
Joint diseases	107	5.0
Pain of the legs resulting from activity	80	3.7
Peripheral vascular disease	7	0.3
Kidney diseases	57	2.7
Schistosomiasis	51	2.4
Hyperthyroid disease	11	0.5
Apoplexy	8	0.4
Malaria	4	0.2
Diabetes mellitus	4	0.2
Cancer	3	0.1
Coronary heart disease	36	1.7
Myocardial infarction	7	0.3
Rheumatic heart disease	8	0.4
Cor pulmonale	4	0.2
Other heart diseases	6	0.3

Fig. 3. Cigarette consumption (number/day)

	Wuhan
Descriptive statistics	
Mean	13.5
Median	10.4
5. – 95. percentile	0 – 30
Minimum-maximum	0 – 50
Correlations (Pearson correlation coefficients for $p<0.01$)	
Age	neg. (– 0.08)
Broca index	neg. (– 0.21)
Blood pressure	neg. (– 0.07)
Heart rate	pos. (0.06)
Alcohol consumption	pos. (0.20)
Alkaline phosphatase	pos. (0.15)
Gamma-GT	n. s.
GPT	n. s.
Triglycerides	neg. (– 0.07)
Cholesterol	n. s.
HDL cholesterol	n. s.
LDL cholesterol	n. s.
VLDL cholesterol	neg. (– 0.09)
Ratio LDL/HDL	n. s.
Uric acid	n. s.
Glucose	n. s.
Frequency distribution (%)	
Wuhan	
Nonsmokers	25.9
Previous smokers	5.5
Total nonsmokers	31.4
1 – 5 cigarettes	5.0
6 – 10 cigarettes	16.9
11 – 20 cigarettes	41.7
21 – 40 cigarettes	3.6
31 – 60 cigarettes	1.1
41 or more cigarettes	0.2

Of the sample population, 13% reported daily sport exercise and another 7.7% reported occasional sport activity. According to the case histories, which included questions about previous serious diseases for which the patient had been medically treated (Table 4), gastrointestinal infections were the most common diseases (16.6%), followed by hepatitis (14.9%). Only seven of 2000 participants reported suffering a myocardial infarction.

The results of the family histories revealed a relatively high percentage of unknown causes of death for the parents (Table 5). In most cases where the causes of death were known, apoplexy resulting from arterial hypertension was found to be the leading factor of death. In contrast, myocardial infarction played a minor role statistically as a cause of death.

Fig. 4. Alcohol consumption (g/day)

	Wuhan
Correlations (Pearson correlation coefficients for p<0.01)	
Age	pos. (0.07)
Broca index	n.s.
Blood pressure	pos. (0.06)
Heart rate	n.s.
Cigarette consumption	pos. (0.20)
Alkaline phosphatase	n.s.
Gamma-GT	pos. (0.16)
GPT	n.s.
Triglycerides	n.s.
Cholesterol	pos. (0.08)
HDL cholesterol	pos. (0.,26)
LDL cholesterol	n.s.
VLDL cholesterol	neg. (−0.07)
Ratio LDL/HDL	neg. (−0.16)
Uric acid	n.s.
Glucose	n.s.
Frequency distribution (%)	
Wuhan	
Alcohol consumption (g/day)	
1 − 10	22.5
11 − 20	12.9
21 − 40	13.8
41 − 60	4.5
61 − 80	0.6
81 − 120	0.1

The evaluation of the results of physical examination shows that for those small in stature (Fig. 7) and low in weight (Fig. 8) there was an average Broca index of 89% (Fig. 9), a value which is acceptable as ideal weight. Undernourished participants were rarely observed.

Despite the relatively high mortality rate from cerebrovascular diseases in China, the average blood pressure value of 121/78 mmHg (Figs. 10, 11) was relatively low compared with the German group. However, in approximately 10% of the cases, an elevated blood pressure of more than 160/95 mmHg was found. A large portion of the participants with known arterial hypertension were not receiving adequate medical treatment (Table 6a + b).

The laboratory results reveal relatively low triglyceride values (Fig. 12). However, a direct comparison with the German group was not possible owing to different withdrawal procedures. Despite adequate fasting periods, 7.35% of the Chinese participants had triglyceride values of over 200 mg/dl, with individual values of up to 900 mg/dl (type IV hyperlipoproteinemia). Lipid electrophoresis revealed type III hyperlipoproteinemia in two cases of elevated triglyceride values.

Striking differences between China and Germany were found for the values of total cholesterol (Fig. 13) and LDL cholesterol (Fig. 14).

Fig. 5. Gamma-glutamyl transpeptidase (Gamma-GT) (U/l)

	Wuhan	Göttingen
Descriptive statistics		
Mean	13.1	23.3
Median	10	15.5
Standard deviation	14.9	28.8
5. – 95. percentile	5 – 30	5 – 65.5
Minimum-maximum	1 – 371	0 – 591

Correlations (Pearson correlation coefficients for $p < 0.01$)

Age	pos. (0.07)
Broca index	pos. (0.17)
Blood pressure	pos. (0.11)
Heart rate	pos. (0.11)
Cigarette consumption	n.s.
Alcohol consumption	pos. (0.16)
Alkaline phosphatase	pos. (0.18)
GPT	pos. (0.23)
Triglycerides	pos. (0.16)
Cholesterol	pos. (0.11)
HDL cholesterol	pos. (0.06)
LDL cholesterol	n.s.
VLDL cholesterol	pos. (0.06)
Ratio LDL/HDL	n.s.
Uric acid	pos. (0.14)
Glucose	pos. (0.09)

Cumulative frequency distribution

Fig. 6. Alkaline phosphatase (U/liter)

	Wuhan	Göttingen
Descriptive statistics		
Mean	127.6	108.4
Median	123	104
Standard deviation	35.1	29.9
5. – 95. percentile	80 – 189	67.8 – 164
Minimum-maximum	16 – 461	47.3 – 352

Correlations (Pearson correlation coefficients for p<0.01)

Age	n.s.
Broca index	n.s.
Blood pressure	n.s.
Heart rate	pos. (0.08)
Cigarette consumption	pos. (0.15)
Alcohol consumption	n.s.
Gamma-GT	pos. (0.18)
GPT	pos. (0.09)
Triglycerides	pos. (0.08)
Cholesterol	n.s.
HDL cholesterol	neg. (−0.10)
LDL cholesterol	n.s.
VLDL cholesterol	pos. (0.06)
Ratio LDL/HDL	pos. (0.06)
Uric acid	n.s.
Glucose	n.s.

Cumulative frequency distribution

Fig. 7. Height (cm)

	Wuhan	Göttingen
Descriptive statistics		
Mean	167.8	174.9
Median	168	175
Standard deviation	5.6	8.9
5. – 95. percentile	159 – 177	165 – 186
Minimum-maximum	145 – 188	– 199

Correlations (Pearson correlation coefficients for $p < 0.01$)

Age	neg. (-0.11)
Broca index	neg. (-0.19)
Blood pressure	n.s.
Heart rate	n.s.
Cigarette consumption	n.s.
Alcohol consumption	n.s.
Alkaline phosphatase	neg. (-0.08)
Gamma-GT	n.s.
GPT	n.s.
Triglycerides	n.s.
Cholesterol	n.s.
HDL cholesterol	n.s.
LDL cholesterol	n.s.
VLDL cholesterol	n.s. -
Ratio LDL/HDL	n.s.
Uric acid	n.s.
Glucose	n.s.

Cumulative frequency distribution

Fig. 8. Weight (kg)

	Wuhan	Göttingen
Descriptive statistics		
Mean	60.5	80.5
Median	60	80
Standard deviation	8.2	11.0
5. – 95. percentile	48 – 76	64 – 99
Minimum-maximum	41 – 96	– 155
Correlations (Pearson correlation coefficients for $p<0.01$)		
Age	n.s.	
Broca index	pos. (0.79)	
Blood pressure	pos. (0.30)	
Heart rate	n.s.	
Cigarette consumption	neg. (-0.18)	
Alcohol consumption	n.s.	
Alkaline phosphatase	neg. (-0.07)	
Gamma-GT	pos. (0.12)	
GPT	pos. (0.06)	
Triglycerides	pos. (0.28)	
Cholesterol	pos. (0.18)	
HDL cholesterol	neg. (-0.26)	
LDL cholesterol	pos. (0.24)	
VLDL cholesterol	pos. (0.28)	
Ratio LDL/HDL	pos. (0.35)	
Uric acid	pos. (0.20)	
Glucose	pos. (0.11)	

Cumulative frequency distribution

Fig. 9. Broca index (%)

	Wuhan	Göttingen
Descriptive statistics		
Mean	89.3	107.4
Median	88	107
Standard deviation	11.1	12.4
5. – 95. percentile	73 – 109	89 – 129
Minimum-maximum	62 – 133	64 – 226
Correlations (Pearson correlation coefficients for p<0.01)		
Age	pos. (0.11)	
Blood pressure	pos. (0.25)	
Heart rate	n.s.	
Cigarette consumption	neg. (-0.21)	
Alcohol consumption	n.s.	
Alkaline phosphatase	n.s.	
Gamma-GT	pos. (0.17)	
GPT	pos. (0.07)	
Triglycerides	pos. (0.32)	
Cholesterol	pos. (0.21)	
HDL cholesterol	neg. (-0.28)	
LDL cholesterol	pos. (0.28)	
VLDL cholesterol	pos. (0.31)	
Ratio LDL/HDL	pos. (0.40)	
Uric acid	pos. (0.21)	
Glucose	pos. (0.11)	

Cumulative frequency distribution

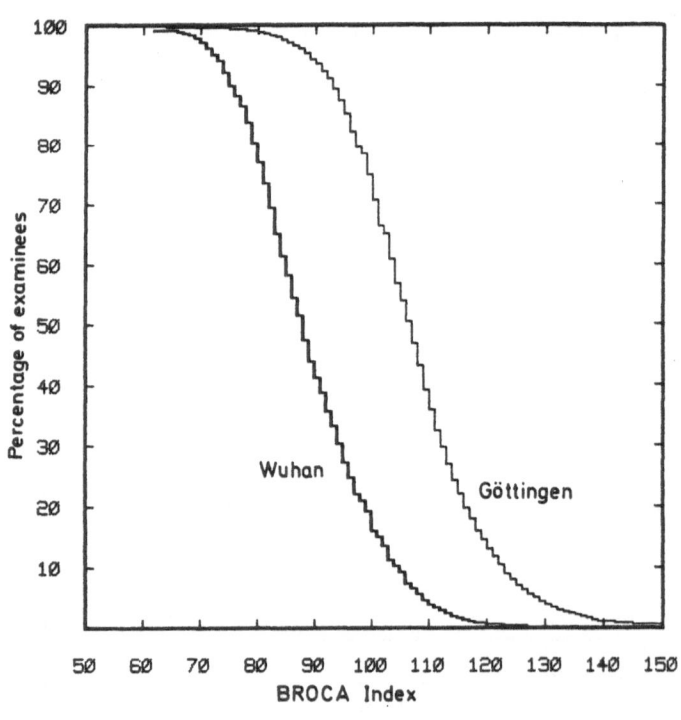

Fig. 10. Systolic blood pressure (mmHg)

	Wuhan	Göttingen
Descriptive statistics		
Mean	120.8	132.0
Median	118	130
Standard deviation	19.3	15.7
5. – 95. percentile	96 – 160	110 – 160
Minimum-maximum	82 – 230	75 – 250

Correlations (Pearson correlation coefficients for $p < 0.01$)

Age	pos. (0.29)
Broca index	pos. (0.25)
Heart rate	pos. (0.09)
Cigarette consumption	neg. (−0.09)
Alcohol consumption	n. s.
Alkaline phosphatase	n. s.
Gamma-GT	pos. (0.11)
GPT	n. s.
Triglycerides	pos. (0.08)
Cholesterol	pos. (0.12)
HDL cholesterol	n. s.
LDL cholesterol	pos. (0.12)
VLDL cholesterol	pos. (0.09)
Ratio LDL/HDL	pos. (0.12)
Uric acid	pos. (0.10)
Glucose	pos. (0.18)

Cumulative frequency distribution

Fig. 11. Diastolic blood pressure (mmHg)

	Wuhan	Göttingen
Descriptive statistics		
Mean	77.6	86.0
Median	80	85
Standard deviation	12.3	9.0
5. – 95. percentile	60 – 100	70 – 100
Minimum-maximum	48 – 146	40 – 160
Correlations (Pearson correlation coefficients for p<0.01)		
Age	pos. (0.20)	
Broca index	pos. (0.30)	
Heart rate	pos. (0.08)	
Cigarette consumption	neg. (− 0.07)	
Alcohol consumption	pos. (0.06)	
Alkaline phosphatase	n.s.	
Gamma-GT	pos. (0.11)	
GPT	n.s.	
Triglycerides	pos. (0.12)	
Cholesterol	pos. (0.16)	
HDL cholesterol	n.s.	
LDL cholesterol	pos. (0.16)	
VLDL cholesterol	pos. (0.12)	
Ratio LDL/HDL	pos. (0.15)	
Uric acid	pos. (0.10)	
Glucose	pos. (0.15)	

Cumulative frequency distribution

Table 5. Cause of death of parents

	Fathers		Mothers	
	(*n*)	(%)	(*n*)	(%)
Apoplexy	221	30.4	187	30.6
Respiratory diseases (including tuberculosis)	192	26.4	124	20.3
Cancer	126	17.3	135	22.1
Accidents/war injuries	108	14.9	58	9.5
Myocardial infarction	22	3.0	21	3.4
Other heart diseases	34	4.7	61	10.0
Arterial hypertension	20	2.8	26	4.2
Diabetes mellitus	4	0.6		
Total	727	100	612	100
Unknown cause of death	938		628	

Table 6a. Arterial hypertension

	(*n*)	(%)
Blood pressure below 160/95 mmHg	1921	89.5
Known hypertension, treated	113	5.3
Known hypertension, not treated	68	3.2
Blood pressure over 160/95 mmHg	227	10.5
Known hypertension, treated	42	2.0
Known hypertension, not treated	59	2.7
Hypertension not known	126	5.9

Table 6b. Diabetes mellitus

	(*n*)	(%)
Blood sugar lower than 120 mg/dl	2127	99.0
Known diabetes, treated	1	0.05
Known diabetes, not treated	0	0
Blood sugar higher than 120 mg/dl	21	0.95
Known diabetes, treated	3	0.15
Known diabetes, not treated	0	0
Diabetes not known	18	0.8

Fig. 12. Triglycerides (mg/dl)

	Wuhan
Descriptive statistics	
Mean	115.2
Median	98
Standard deviation	70.0
5. – 95. percentile	57 – 228
Minimum-maximum	21 – 864

Correlations (Pearson correlation coefficients for p<0.01)

Age	n. s.
Broca index	pos. (0.32)
Blood pressure	pos. (0.08)
Heart rate	n. s.
Cigarette consumption	neg. (-0.07)
Alcohol consumption	n. s.
Alkaline phosphatase	pos. (0.08)
Gamma-GT	pos. (0.16)
GPT	pos. (0.06)
Cholesterol	pos. (0.32)
HDL cholesterol	neg. (0.23)
LDL cholesterol	pos. (0.17)
VLDL cholesterol	pos. (0.79)
Ratio LDL/HDL	pos. (0.29)
Uric acid	pos. (0.16)
Glucose	pos. (0.18)

Cumulative frequency distribution

Fig. 13. Cholesterol (mg/dl)

	Wuhan	Göttingen
Descriptive statistics		
Mean	154.9	217.3
Median	153.5	214
Standard deviation	27.4	39.8
5. – 95. percentile	113 – 202	159 – 286
Minimum-maximum	80 – 289	95 – 499

Correlations (Pearson correlation coefficients for $p<0.01$)	
Age	pos. (0.11)
Broca index	pos. (0.21)
Blood pressure	pos. (0.12)
Heart rate	n.s.
Cigarette consumption	n.s.
Alcohol consumption	pos. (0.08)
Alkaline phosphatase	n.s.
Gamma-GT	pos. (0.11)
GPT	n.s.
Triglycerides	pos. (0.32)
HDL cholesterol	pos. (0,37)
LDL cholesterol	pos. (0.88)
VLDL cholesterol	pos. (0.33)
Ratio LDL/HDL	pos. (0.38)
Uric acid	pos. (0.07)
Glucose	pos. (0.15)

Cumulative frequency distribution

Fig. 14. Beta-(LDL)-Cholesterol (mg/dl) as determined by lipidelectrophoresis [12]

	Wuhan	Göttingen
Descriptive statistics		
Mean	94.4	144.8
Median	92.6	142.0
Standard deviation	22.8	33.4
5. – 95. percentile	61.4 – 135.7	95.9 – 204.0
Minimum-maximum	37.0 – 195.8	46.3 – 381.0

Correlations (Pearson correlation coefficients for $p < 0.01$)	
Age	pos. (0.10)
Broca index	pos. (0.28)
Blood pressure	pos. (0.12)
Heart rate	n.s.
Cigarette consumption	n.s.
Alcohol consumption	n.s.
Alkaline phosphatase	n.s.
Gamma-GT	n.s.
GPT	n.s.
Triglycerides	pos. (0.17)
Cholesterol	pos. (0.88)
HDL cholesterol	n.s.
VLDL cholesterol	pos. (0.13)
Ratio LDL/HDL	pos. (0.69)
Uric acid	pos. (0.10)
Glucose	pos. (0.11)

Cumulative frequency distribution

Fig. 15. Alpha-(HDL)cholesterol (mg/dl) as determined by lipidelectrophoresis [12]

	Wuhan	Göttingen
Descriptive statistics		
Mean	49.5	48.4
Median	48.2	47.7
Standard deviation	11.9	11.8
5. – 95. percentile	32.2 – 70.7	30.7 – 69.0
Minimum-maximum	17.8 – 121.0	13.4 – 108.0

Correlations (Pearson correlation coefficients for p<0.01)

Age	pos. (0.07)
Broca index	neg. (−0.20)
Blood pressure	n.s. (0.12)
Heart rate	n.s.
Cigarette consumption	n.s.
Alcohol consumption	pos. (0.26)
Alkaline phosphatase	neg. (−0.10)
Gamma-GT	pos. (0.06)
GPT	n.s.
Triglycerides	neg. (−0.23)
Cholesterol	pos. (0.37)
LDL cholesterol	n.s.
VLDL cholesterol	neg. (−0.23)
Ratio LDL/HDL	neg. (−0.65)
Uric acid	neg. (−0.12)
Glucose	n.s.

Cumulative frequency distribution

Fig. 16. Ratio LDL-cholesterol/HDL-cholesterol as determined by lipidelectrophoresis [12]

	Wuhan
Descriptive statistics	
Mean	2.0
Median	1.9
Standard deviation	0.7
5.–95. percentile	1.1–3.4
Minimum-maximum	0.9–7.2
Correlations (Pearson correlation coefficients for p<0.01)	
Age	n.s.
Broca index	pos. (0.40)
Blood pressure	pos. (0.12)
Heart rate	n.s.
Cigarette consumption	n.s.
Alcohol consumption	neg. (−0.16)
Alkaline phosphatase	pos. (0.06)
Gamma-GT	n.s.
GPT	pos. (0.07)
Triglycerides	pos. (0.29)
Cholesterol	pos. (0.38)
HDL cholesterol	neg. (−0.65)
LDL cholesterol	pos. (0.69)
VLDL cholesterol	pos. (0.26)
Uric acid	pos. (0.16)
Glucose	pos. (0.07)

Cumulative frequency distribution

Fig. 17. Praebeta-(VLDL)-Cholesterol (mg/dl) as determined by lipidelectrophoresis [12]

	Wuhan	Göttingen
Descriptive statistics		
Mean	11.0	23.6
Median	9.0	19.9
Standard deviation	8.8	17.1
5. – 95. percentile	3.0 – 26.0	6.6 – 50.2
Minimum-maximum	0.6 – 90.7	1.3 – 310.0
Correlations (Pearson correlation coefficients for $p < 0.01$)		
Age	n. s.	
Broca index	pos. (0.31)	
Blood pressure	pos. (0.09)	
Heart rate	n. s.	
Cigarette consumption	neg. (– 0.09)	
Alcohol consumption	neg. (– 0.07)	
Alkaline phosphatase	pos. (0.06)	
Gamma-GT	n. s.	
GPT	n. s.	
Triglycerides	pos. (0.79)	
Cholesterol	pos. (0.33)	
HDL cholesterol	neg. (– 0.23)	
LDL cholesterol	pos. (0.13)	
Ratio LDL/HDL	pos. (0.26)	
Uric acid	pos. (0.15)	
Glucose	pos. (0.10)	

Cumulative frequency distribution

Fig. 18. Uric acid (mg/dl)

	Wuhan	Göttingen
Descriptive statistics		
Mean	4.7	6.1
Median	4.7	6.0
Standard deviation	1.0	1.1
5. – 95. percentile	3.2 – 6.4	4.1 – 8.3
Minimum-maximum	1.8 – 12.0	1.1 – 13.7

Correlations (Pearson correlation coefficients for $p<0.01$)	
Age	pos. (0.07)
Broca index	pos. (0.21)
Blood pressure	pos. (0.10)
Heart rate	n.s.
Cigarette consumption	n.s.
Alcohol consumption	n.s.
Alkaline phosphatase	n.s.
Gamma-GT	pos. (0.14)
GPT	n.s.
Triglycerides	pos. (0.16)
Cholesterol	pos. (0.07)
HDL cholesterol	neg. (-0.12)
LDL cholesterol	pos. (0.10)
VLDL cholesterol	pos. (0.15)
Ratio LDL/HDL	pos. (0.16)
Glucose	n.s.

Cumulative frequency distribution

Fig. 19. Glucose (mg/dl)

	Wuhan	Göttingen
Descriptive statistics		
Mean	86.7	113.1
Median	86	107
Standard deviation	14.4	32.2
5.–95. percentile	69–104	
Minimum-maximum	37–349	32–507

Correlations (Pearson correlation coefficients for p<0.01)	
Age	pos. (0.09)
Broca index	pos. (0.11)
Blood pressure	pos. (0.18)
Heart rate	n.s.
Cigarette consumption	n.s.
Alcohol consumption	n.s.
Alkaline phosphatase	n.s.
Gamma-GT	pos. (0.09)
GPT	n.s.
Triglycerides	pos. (0.18)
Cholesterol	pos. (0.15)
HDL cholesterol	n.s.
LDL cholesterol	pos. (0.11)
VLDL cholesterol	pos. (0.10)
Ratio LDL/HDL	pos. (0.07)
Uric acid	n.s.

Cumulative frequency distribution

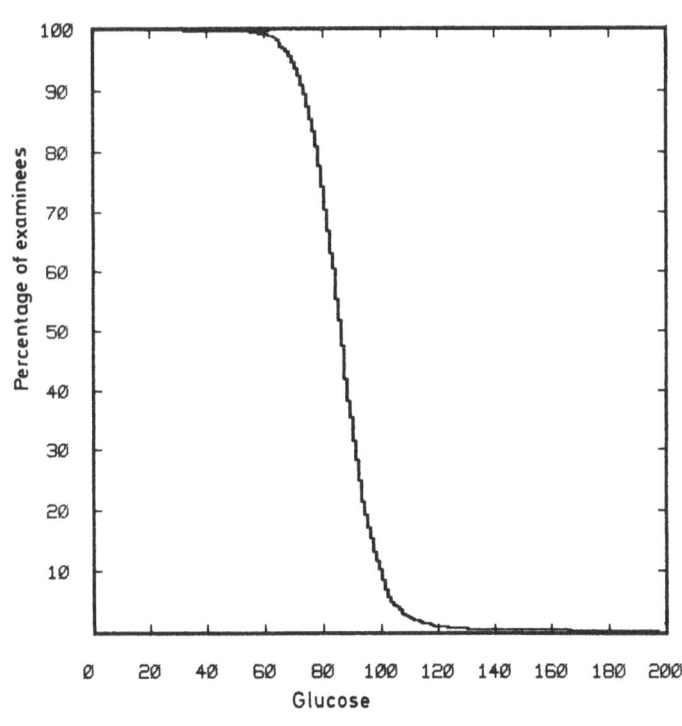

Fig. 20. Glutamate pyruvate transaminase (GPT) (U/liter)

	Wuhan	Göttingen
Descriptive statistics		
Mean	19.2	15.6
Median	16	14
Standard deviation	15.8	8.7
5. – 95. percentile	7 – 41	7 – 29.1
Minimum-maximum	2 – 510	1.5 – 178

Correlations (Pearson correlation coefficients for $p<0.01$)	
Age	n. s.
Broca index	pos. (0.07)
Blood pressure	n. s.
Heart rate	n. s.
Cigarette consumption	n. s.
Alcohol consumption	n. s.
Alkaline phosphatase	pos. (0.09)
Gamma-GT	pos. (0.23)
Triglycerides	pos. (0.06)
Cholesterol	n. s.
HDL cholesterol	n. s.
LDL cholesterol	n. s.
VLDL cholesterol	n. s.
Ratio LDL/HDL	pos. (0.07)
Uric acid	n. s.
Glucose	n. s.

Cumulative frequency distribution

Table 7. Comparison of the risk indicators for Wuhan and Göttingen

	Wuhan		Göttingen	
	mean	S.D.	mean	S.D.
Cholesterol (mg/dl)	155	27	217	40
LDL Cholesterol (mg/dl)	95	23	145	33
HDL Cholesterol (mg/dl)	49	12	48	12
VLDL Cholesterol (mg/dl)	11	9	24	17
Uric acid (mg/dl)	4.7	1.0	6.1	1.1
Broca index (%)	89	11	107	12
Blood pressure, systolic (mmHg)	121	19	132	16
Blood pressure, diastolic (mmHg)	78	12	86	9
Apolipoprotein A − I (mg/dl)	107	27	125	32
Apolipoprotein B (mg/dl)	79	14	121	26

These results verified earlier studies in China [5]. The HDL cholesterol values were found to be within the same range as in the German study (Fig. 15), although the total cholesterol values in China were low. These results in China reveal a very favorable LDL/HDL quotient (Fig. 16), which represents a specific risk indicator (atherosclerosis index). Accordingly, the values for apoprotein B, the major protein constituent of LDL, were relatively low, whereas the values for the major protein components of HDL, apoprotein A-I and A-II, show no significant differences from the results of the German study (Table 7). VLDL cholesterol levels were also lower in the Chinese than in the German group (Fig. 17).

The uric acid value (Fig. 18), a further important metabolic parameter and risk indicator, is significantly lower in China than in Germany. The serum glucose values are almost exclusively within the normal range (Fig. 19). The rate of known diabetes mellitus is extremely low (Table 4).

A high percentage of the Chinese participants showed elevated GPT activity (Fig. 20). This finding corresponds with a high incidence of hepatitis A and B. Of the investigated participants, 21% were HBs positive, and 95% had antibodies against hepatitis B. A significant correlation between GPT and HDL cholesterol was not found, so that hepatitis-related liver disease was unable to account for the relative high HDL cholesterol values.

The evaluation of the correlations between the other risk parameters showed a specifically positive correlation between body weight, blood pressure, triglycerides, total cholesterol, LDL and very-low-density lipoprotein (VLDL) cholesterol, uric acid, and serum glucose. There are negative correlation coefficients between HDL cholesterol on the one hand and body weight, triglycerides, VLDL cholesterol, and uric acid on the other hand.

Table 8. Influence of cigarette consumption (mean)

Cigarettes per day (n)	0	1 – 5	6 – 10	11 – 20	More than 20	Exsmokers
(n)	509	125	309	838	196	169
Weight (kg)	62	62	61	59	59	64
Broca index (%)	92	92	89	87	88	94
Blood pressure, systolic (mmHg)	123	118	122	119	121	125
Blood pressure diastolic (mmHg)	79	76	78	76	78	81
Triglycerides (mg/dl)	123	110	115	107	123	128
Cholesterol (mg/dl)	157	152	154	154	155	160
Alpha-cholesterol (HDL, mg/dl)	49	50	50	50	49	47
Beta-cholesterol (LDL, mg/dl)	95	92	93	94	95	100
Praebeta-cholesterol (VLDL, mg/dl)	12	10	11	10	11	12
Ratio LDL/HDL cholesterol	2.1	1.9	2.0	2.0	2.0	2.2
Alkaline phosphatase (U/liter)	121	120	126	132	136	125
Gamma-GT (U/liter)	12	12	13	12	16	16
GPT (U/liter)	20	17	20	19	18	20
Uric acid (mg/dl)	4.7	4.8	4.7	4.7	4.8	4.9
Glucose (mg/dl)	88	86	86	86	87	86
Cardialgia (%)	25	33	17	26	21	19

Influence of Life Style

The individual life habits which exert a predominant influence on risk for cardiovascular disease are the degree of physical activity during labor or sports, cigarette smoking, and consumption of alcohol. Table 8 shows the influence of cigarette smoking. The body weight of nonsmokers is slightly above that of smokers. Exsmokers seem to compensate for former smoking habits by increasing food intake. Data for blood pressure, serum triglyceride, and serum cholesterol parallel those for body weight. In contrast, there is no correlation between cigarette smoking and HDL cholesterol. The other parameters in Table 8 also show no correlation with smoking habits.

As expected, consumption of alcohol (Table 9) increases serum gamma-GT significantly. Total serum cholesterol and HDL cholesterol levels are higher in alcohol consumers, but there is no difference in LDL cholesterol levels between drinkers and nondrinkers.

Table 9. Influence of alcohol consumption (mean)

Alcohol consumption (g/day)	0	1 – 20	21 – 40	41 – 60	over 60
(*n*)	974	764	298	82	30
Weight (kg)	60	60	60	61	62
Broca index (%)	90	89	89	91	93
Blood pressure, systolic (mmHg)	121	120	122	124	125
Blood pressure, diastolic (mmHg)	77	77	78	80	82
Triglycerides (mg/dl)	118	110	117	126	100
Cholesterol (mg/dl)	154	154	160	159	161
Alpha-cholesterol (HDL, mg/dl)	47	49	54	58	58
Beta-cholesterol (LDL, mg/dl)	95	94	95	90	93
Praebeta-cholesterol (VLDL, mg/dl)	12	10	10	11	9
Ratio LDL/HDL cholesterol	2.1	2.0	1.9	1.6	1.7
Alkaline phosphatase (U/liter)	130	125	126	127	125
Gamma-GT (U/liter)	12	12	15	26	18
GPT (U/liter)	21	18	17	16	27
Uric acid (mg/dl)	4.7	4.7	4.7	4.9	4.6
Glucose (mg/dl)	86	87	88	88	84
Cardialgia (%)	25	21	21	24	13

Increased relative body weight, expressed as the Broca index (quotient of body weight in kg to height in cm minus 100), has a strong unfavorable effect on all investigated serum lipid parameters, as well as on blood pressure, serum uric acid, and glucose levels (Table 10). Furthermore, overweight participants reported angina pectoris episodes more often than normal weight participants.

The degree of physical work has a strong influence on the parameters studied (Table 11). Although Chinese workers performing heavy physical labor get bonuses for food rations, increased physical labor correlated negatively with body weight. Triglycerides, total cholesterol, and LDL and VLDL cholesterol display similar tendencies. In addition, those who perform heavy physical labor have the highest HDL cholesterol levels, and therefore the most favorable risk factor profiles with respect to the development of atherosclerosis. In contrast, the cadre groups have the most unfavorable risk factor profiles. Members of this group do not usually perform heavy labor, and in many cases, have the opportunity to use motor vehicles. Furthermore, their food rations are higher, and their daily caloric intake often exceeds their daily energy requirements. As a consequence their

Table 10. Influence of relative body weight (mean)

Broca index (%)	under 80	81 – 90	91 – 100	101 – 110	over 110
(n)	422	787	512	326	86
Blood pressure, systolic (mmHg)	115	119	122	128	133
Blood pressure, diastolic (mmHg)	73	76	79	83	87
Triglycerides (mg/dl)	92	104	118	147	182
Cholesterol (mg/dl)	149	151	157	163	169
Alpha-cholesterol (HDL, mg/dl)	54	51	48	45	41
Beta-cholesterol (LDL, mg/dl)	87	91	97	103	109
Praebeta-cholesterol (VLDL, mg/dl)	8	10	12	15	18
Ratio LDL/HDL cholesterol	1.7	1.9	2.1	2.4	2.8
Alkaline phosphatase (U/liter)	133	125	126	128	132
Gamma-GT (U/liter)	11	12	13	17	21
GPT (U/liter)	19	18	20	20	22
Uric acid (mg/dl)	4.5	4.6	4.7	5.0	5.3
Glucose (mg/dl)	84	86	88	87	91
Cardialgia (%)	21	21	26	25	28

values for body weight, blood pressure, triglycerides, total cholesterol, and LDL and VLDL cholesterol were higher than those of the laborers, and their HDL cholesterol levels were lower. The group of medical doctors had a risk profile similar to that of the cadre group. Both groups reported angina pectoris symptoms more often than the others.

Sport activities have almost no effect on the risk factor parameters in this Chinese population sample (Table 12), possibly because physical activity is relatively high even without sports, and the Chinese group in general has a very favorable risk factor profile.

Conclusion

The incidence and mortality from coronary heart disease and myocardial infarction in China are much lower than in Germany or in other Western industrialized countries. In order to gain more insight into these differences, the levels of the major established coronary risk factors in both countries were compared. In 2000

Table 11. Influence of physical labor (mean)

	Heavy physical labor	Medium-heavy physical labor	Light- physical labor	Cadres	Physicians
(n)	337	1233	523	32	15
Weight (kg)	60	60	61	67	65
Broca-index (%)	89	89	90	97	95
Blood pressure, systolic (mmHg)	124	119	121	135	132
Blood pressure, diastolic (mmHg)	79	77	77	78	85
Triglycerides (mg/dl)	104	114	122	139	144
Cholesterol (mg/dl)	153	154	157	166	182
Alpha-cholesterol (HDL, mg/dl)	50	50	49	48	50
Beta-cholesterol (LDL, mg/dl)	93	93	97	104	115
Praebeta-cholesterol (VLDL, mg/dl)	9	11	11	14	16
Ratio LDL/HDL cholesterol	2.0	2.0	2.1	2.3	2.4
Alkaline phos-phatase (U/liter)	132	127	126	127	112
Gamma-GT (U/liter)	13	12	14	25	17
GPT (U/liter)	22	18	20	16	19
Uric acid (mg/dl)	4.3	4.8	4.8	5.0	5.0
Glucose (mg/dl)	90	86	86	91	86
Cardialgia (%)	20	22	25	47	40

Table 12. Influence of sport activities (mean)

	Sport activities			
	Every day	2–4 times per week	1 time per week	No sports
(n)	279	101	65	1701
Weight (kg)	63	60	61	60
Broca index (%)	91	89	89	89
Blood pressure, systolic (mmHg)	124	121	124	120
Blood pressure, diastolic (mmHg)	79	77	80	77
Triglycerides (mg/dl)	119	104	114	115
Cholesterol (mg/dl)	157	155	158	154
Alpha-cholesterol (HDL, mg/dl)	50	50	51	49
Beta-cholesterol (LDL, mg/dl)	96	95	97	94
Praebeta-cholesterol (VLDL, mg/dl)	11	10	11	11
Ratio LDL/HDL cholesterol	2.0	2.0	2.0	2.0
Alkaline phosphatase (U/liter)	130	123	124	128
Gamma-GT (U/liter)	14	13	17	13
GPT (U/liter)	19	19	28	19
Uric acid (mg/dl)	4.8	4.8	4.6	4.7
Glucose (mg/dl)	87	87	88	87
Cardialgia (%)	25	24	14	23

Chinese male workers aged 40–60 years, a mean serum cholesterol level of 155 mg/dl was found, which is much lower than in a similar German population. This difference was found only for LDL and VLDL fractions. Almost no difference between Chinese and Germans was found for HDL cholesterol levels. Serum uric acid levels and weight indices were also lower in the Chinese population. In a subgroup of the participants, a nutritional assessment was carried out. Total caloric intake was as high as in the German workers, but fat content was much lower and carbohydrate consumption higher. The daily cholesterol intake in the Chinese is only one-third that usually consumed by adult German males.

Acknowledgements

We thank M. Mao, G. Zhang, S. Sun, H. He and L. Cao for contributing to this work. The project was supported by the Deutsche Forschungsgemeinschaft and the Deutscher Akademischer Austauschdienst, Bonn.

References

1. Statistisches Bundesamt Wiesbaden (1984) Statistisches Jahrbuch 1983 für die Bundesrepublik Deutschland. Kohlhammer, Stuttgart
2. Schettler G (1980) Pathophysiologie, Klinik und prognostische Bedeutung der Hyperlipoproteinämien. Dtsch. Ärzteblatt 77:661
3. Wilson PW, Garrison RJ, Castelli WP, Feinleib M, McNamara PM, Kannel WB (1980) Prevalence of coronary heart disease in the Framingham offspring study: Role of lipoprotein cholesterols. Am J Cardiol 46:649
4. Wuhan Medical College (1982), personal information
5. State Statistical Bureau, PRC (1983) Statistical Yearbook of China 1981. Economic Information & Agency , Hong Kong
6. Chen H, Zhuang H, Han Q (1983) Serum high density lipoprotein cholesterol and factors influencing its level in healthy Chinese. Atherosclerosis 48:71
7. Kesteloot H, Huang DX, Yang XSh, Claes J, Rosseneu M, Geboers J, Joossens JV (1985) Serum lipids in the People's Republic of China: Comparison of western and eastern populations. Arteriosclerosis 5:427
8. Seidel D, Cremer P (1986) Die Bedeutung von Lebensalter, relativem Körpergewicht, Rauchgewohnheiten und Alkoholgenuß für die Häufigkeit atherogener Fettstoffwechselmuster. Lebensversicherungsmedizin 11:54
9. Wieland H, Seidel D (1983) A simple specific method for precipitation of low density lipoproteins. J Lipid Res 24:904
10. Siedel J, Schlumberger H, Klose S, Ziegenhorn J, Wahlefeld AW (1981) Improved reagent for the enzymatic determination of serum cholesterol. J Clin Chem Clin Biochem 19:838
11. Weinstock N, Bartholome M, Seidel D (1981) Determination of apolipoprotein A1 by kinetic nephelometry. Biochim Biophys Acta 663:279
12. Wieland H, Cremer P, Seidel D (1982) Determination of apolipoprotein B by kinetic immuno-nephelometry. J Lipid Res 23:893
13. Wieland H, Seidel D (1978) Fortschritte in der Analytik des Lipoproteinmusters. Innere Med 5:290
14. Burnstein M, Samaille J (1960) Sur un dosage du cholestérol lié aux α- et aux β-lipoprotéines du sérum. Clin Chim Acta 5:609
15. Bachorik PS, Wood PD, Albers JJ, Steiner P, Dempsey M, Kuba K, Warnick R, Karlsson L (1976) Plasma high-density lipoprotein cholesterol concentrations determined after removal of other lipoproteins by heparin-manganese precipitation or by ultracentrifugation. Clin Chem 22:1828
16. Friedewald WF, Levy RI, Frederikson DS (1972) Estimation of LDL-cholesterol concentration without use of the preparative ultracentrifuge. Clin Chem 18:499
17. SAS Institute, Inc. (1985) SAS User's guide: statistics, version 5 edition. SAS Institute, Inc., Cary NC, pp 1 – 956